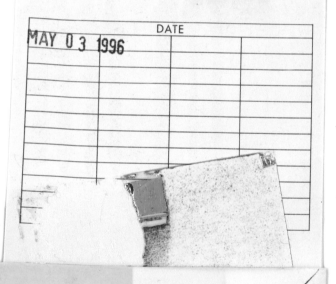

THE
FIVE
OF
ME

THE FIVE OF ME

The Autobiography of a Multiple Personality

Henry Hawksworth
with Ted Schwarz

Introduction by Ralph Allison, M. D.

Henry Regnery Company · Chicago

921
Hawks

Library of Congress Cataloging in Publication Data

Hawksworth, Henry.
   The five of me.

   1. Multiple personality—Biography.   2. Hawks-
worth, Henry.   I. Schwarz, Theodore, joint author.
II. Title.
RC569.5.M8H38   1977   616.8′523 [B]   76-55662
ISBN 0-8092-7869-3

Published by Henry Regnery Company
180 North Michigan Avenue, Chicago, Illinois 60601
Manufactured in the United States of America
Library of Congress Catalog Card Number: 76-55662
International Standard Book Number: 0-8092-7869-3

Published simultaneously in Canada by
Beaverbooks
953 Dillingham Road
Pickering, Ontario L1W 1Z7
Canada

Introduction

The story you are about to read is true. Henry Hawksworth is one of over thirty patients I have treated for the rarely reported phenomenon known as multiple personality.

My first encounter with this unusual psychological problem came in 1972 after ten years of practice in general psychiatry. Multiple personality is a condition in which the patient's mind divides into two or more unique personalities who act independently of each other. This condition was extensively studied by Dr. Morton Prince of Boston in the early part of the twentieth century. His classic description of eight years of treatment of Miss Beauchamp was published in 1913 under the title *The Dissociation of a Personality*. Subsequent case histories were published by H. H. Goddard (*Two Souls in One Body?*, 1927) and S. I. Franz (*Persons I and III*, 1933). Then in 1957 Drs. Thigpen and Cleckley wrote *The Three Faces of Eve*, which was made into an Academy Award-winning movie. More recently, *Sybil*, by Flora Schreiber, has been a best seller.

Since then Dr. Robert Stoller wrote about his very strange patient in *Splitting: A Case of Female Masculinity*. But none of these studies were about men, a rarity in this field, in which only about fifteen percent of the few cases reported have been males.

In my own practice, I had treated a number of women with this disorder, but no males. Before Mr. Hawksworth arrived at the door of my office, I had seen two men with this condition for legal evaluations only and one man for short-term in-patient treatment. This last man was so difficult to cope with that I was unable to treat him on an out-patient basis. So when along came Henry and his "friends," Dana, Johnny, Peter, and Phil, I had had some preparation. But he still had a storehouse of surprises for me. For when such radically different individuals all inhabit one body, how can one be truly prepared for the strange experiences sure to come?

During the previous years in which I had been learning about men and women with multiple personalities, I had come to realize that, to create this very strange phenomenon, there had to be certain interrelating factors existing. First, these children arrive in this life with an inability to learn from experience, leading to failure to integrate everyday incidences into their general body of knowledge. Next, they are in a moral limbo, unwilling to decide whether to be good or bad, straddling the fence on all ethical issues. Then, they are born into a body with an especially sensitive nervous system, one that is as attuned to the emotional outpourings of others as an albino is to the rays of the sun. Lastly, they are born into a family constellation where polarity is encouraged and fostered and where they are forced to take sides, without ever being sure of which side to take. To accommodate both sides, they have to split their minds while still, themselves, sitting on the fence.

Family life factors usually include being an unwanted child and then being caught in the pull of love-hate between father and mother. The favored parent, seen as the only loving one, often leaves the home before the child is old enough to go to school. Skeletons in the family closet are regarded as secrets to be shamefully kept from all intruders. Fun may be looked down upon, especially if it is related to sexual activity. In girls, the first sexual experience is usually traumatic, a rape or child molestation, with subsequent shame and self-condemnation.

In most cases, the existence of multiple personalities goes unnoticed by doctors treating the patient. My first case involved a woman who was hospitalized in a psychiatric ward where the staff refused to admit to the existence of more than one personality controlling the woman's body. The alter-personality was infuriated with the hospital staff for ignoring her. She decided that she was not going to bother taking control of the body so long as no one would speak to her. She remained in the recesses of the patient's mind until she was released as "cured." Then, when the patient left the hospital, she started taking control for varying periods of time, and the patient began having as many problems as she had encountered before entering the ward.

Many times the patient's problem is misdiagnosed. There is a condition, known as manic-depressive illness, in whch the patient experiences radical shifts in mood for no apparent reason. He or she can be laughing gaily one day, then sobbing endless tears the next, although nothing funny or sad has happened. When it is assumed that a multiple personality is a manic-depressive, the patient is treated accordingly. Naturally, the treatment fails to work, for the simple reason that the two are not the same condition.

Henry Hawksworth's case is a graphic example of how the condition of multiple personality can create a horror-filled nightmare situation for the person suffering from it. One of his personalities, Peter, was a seven-year-old child living in a forty-year-old man's body. He enjoyed going to amusement parks and writing poetry, climbing trees and smelling flowers—all during periods when another personality, Dana, was supposed to be working as a highly paid corporate executive.

The very worst was Johnny, a violent sociopath who attempted murder several times when still a child. As an adult, he would tear apart bars, single-handedly take on an entire motorcycle gang, and beat women during wild sexual escapades—all while Dana was living a quiet life as a devoted family man who knew nothing of this other's existence.

The treatment of Henry's condition took almost two years after he first came to see me. Several weeks passed before I became aware of his alter-personalities and realized just how serious a problem I had encountered.

Today, Henry Hawksworth is an integrated, productive individual. He is able to experience a full range of emotions; the violent rage that was Johnny is no longer a part of him. The story that follows tells of his forty-year search for his own identity and of the lives of the personalities who regularly controlled his body. It is unusual, often shocking, and all true. He is a courageous man who was able to face a horrible truth about himself and, with the aid of psychotherapy, triumph over it.

Ralph B. Allison, M. D.

CHAPTER 1

One afternoon when I was three years old, I lay down to take my nap. I didn't awaken for forty years. No one knew I was sleeping, because during that time four different people took my place.

I was a multiple personality.

My problem might have gone unnoticed if Dana, the first and most pervasive of my other personalities, had been the only person anyone encountered. He was a serious, unemotional child whose interests were centered on books, much to the disgust of his athletically oriented father. Dana as a child built an elaborate home chemistry lab and enjoyed studying astronomy. His grades were frequently high and he eventually qualified for the U.S. Naval Academy. As an adult he turned his skills to the business world and held executive jobs that paid as much as $4,000 a month.

Unfortunately, every time Dana's life seemed to reach a high point, Johnny, the second of my hidden personalities, would do something to get him fired. For example, there was that warm spring afternoon in 1970 when Dana was finishing his day's work at the health club he managed. He had recently completed his initial training period and the owner had been so impressed that he decided to give Dana full executive status at once, a position others had worked years to achieve. His paycheck that day included a substantial raise, plus a bonus.

"Ann?" Dana said to his wife on the telephone. "Don't bother to fix dinner tonight. Something wonderful's happened and I'm taking you out to celebrate."

"What is it?" she asked.

"I'll tell you when I pick you up. Just be waiting in your best dress."

He was smiling as he climbed into his car, started the engine, and eased out into traffic. He was always a careful driver, well aware of how dangerous California traffic could be.

Then without warning he suddenly became depressed. For two or three seconds he felt as if he were sinking into a black pit, whirling ever downward. His body slumped and he lost consciousness.

Then in a moment the body jerked erect once more. Johnny had taken control. His lip curled slightly and his eyes narrowed. His foot stabbed at the accelerator and he began weaving in and out, hurling the car into any opening in the traffic that he could find. There was a supermarket up ahead where Dana was known by the manager. He pulled into the lot and got out of the car.

Johnny's walk was heavy. His footsteps thumped against the tile floor of the supermarket as he made his way to the manager's office. On the way he made an obscene remark to an attractive girl in a halter top, waiting with an overloaded shopping cart in the check-out line.

Johnny faked Dana's signature as best he could. Their handwriting was not the same, but there was enough similarity so that the manager didn't suspect anything. Be-

sides, the manager had seen Dana many times before; he
had no reason to refuse the check.

San Jose seemed the best place to have a little fun.
Johnny drove quickly, his thoughts suddenly on Ann. She
would be waiting for Dana's arrival, he knew. But Dana
was gone. That bitch he married could stand around all
night for all Johnny cared. Broads were all right for a one-
night stand, but he wasn't about to marry one. Furthermore, he'd be damned if he'd call Ann to tell her Dana
wouldn't be coming. She'd have to figure that one out for
herself.

He began bar-hopping, looking for action, seldom staying in any one place long enough to have more than a
drink or two. By 1 A.M. he was feeling good—a little drunk
perhaps, but still game, still anxious for a little more fun.
San Jose, however, was already closing up for the night
like the hick town it was. That meant he would have to
move on to Los Angeles. He called the airport to book a
flight.

"I'm sorry, Sir," said the person on the other end of the
telephone. "There are no more scheduled flights until nine
tomorrow morning. If you'd care to make a reservation for
that. . . ."

Shove it, thought Johnny. He still had plenty of money.
He'd drive out to the airport and see if he could charter a
flight.

The private pilot Johnny found at the airport was tired,
but for $125 he thought he could find the energy to make
the flight. They arrived in L. A. at 4:30 A.M. and Johnny
immediately checked into a hotel room, the drinks and the
late hour finally catching up with him. He soon fell into a
deep sleep.

Before he could waken from the nap, Peter—the third of
my other personalities—took over.

Peter leaped from the bed, his baby face radiating happiness. He looked in the mirror at the clothing Dana and
Johnny had been wearing and laughed at the way he was

dressed. Dana had no taste, that was for certain. But there was still plenty of money left from the large check that Dana had received that day. Buying something else with a little more style would be no problem.

"Good morning," he chirped happily to the motel manager as he headed for the lobby door. His high-pitched voice seemed strange, coming from a six-foot man's body. His peculiar walk, too, caused several people to turn and stare at him. He rose lightly on his toes with each step, his body bobbing down the street like a happy jack-in-the-box. He seemed to radiate love for every person he passed.

Peter walked five miles before reaching the downtown area. He searched until he found a department store that carried the kind of clothing he wanted. His new pants were bright blue, a pleasant contrast to the multi-colored, striped polo shirt he had instantly fallen in love with. He added some pointed-toe shoes with shining buckles and a long string of beads to wear around his neck. When he left, he was so pleased with his new look that he didn't even bother to take his old clothes with him, leaving them on a hook in the dressing room.

Outside the sun was shining and its warmth penetrated his body, seeming to add to the glow that always radiated from within him. Following the directions he received from a bemused stranger, he boarded a bus and rode to the Venice beach.

There he walked along the boardwalk area, stopping once at a penny arcade to watch someone play a pinball machine. He stopped also at a refreshment stand and bought popcorn and cotton candy. Then he wandered happily to the water's edge.

Sitting on the moist sand, he began to shape a small mound, then another and another. Soon a slightly lopsided sand castle, complete with moat, appeared in the sand. The tide was moving in. He finished the structure just as the water began lapping at the castle door. Then he watched while wave after wave slowly battered his creation down. His pants grew wet from the water and his new shoes were filled with sand; he didn't care.

Constructing the sand castle had given him an appetite. A hot dog was what he wanted, he decided. Then he discovered that he had only a few cents in his pocket. Dana's wallet, he suddenly remembered, was still in the pair of pants he had abandoned in the department store. He would have to find a way to earn some money if he was going to eat.

He returned to the boardwalk and entered the first bar he found—an old, weather-beaten building with peeling paint and wood pitted from the wind and salt air. Inside it was quite dark. He had to stand in the entrance a few moments until his eyes could adjust to the reduced light. Then he made his way across the sawdust floor to the aged oak bar at the back of the room. Several rows of liquor bottles were lined on shelves behind the bar, beneath decorative fishing nets, sea shells, and a huge fish tank filled with exotic saltwater fish. The bartender was dressed as a seaman, with an open-necked shirt, bell-bottom Levi's, and an ancient Navy cap cocked at the back of his head.

Peter immediately liked the atmosphere of the place.

He walked over to the bar and climbed up on one of the stools.

"What'll you have?" asked the bartender.

And without even seeming to think about it, Peter suddenly had a plan. He would analyze the bartender's handwriting, he suggested, in exchange for a beer and two hard-boiled eggs. His eyes as he made the suggestion were wide, and he was grinning broadly.

The bartender hesitated a moment. But Peter looked so sincere—perhaps even a bit simple-minded—that he couldn't resist him. He agreed to the terms.

He wrote his name and a few facts about himself on a piece of paper, then handed it to Peter, who immediately told him what the loops and letter formations revealed. Peter had had no scientific training in Graphoanalysis; he was simply combining guesswork, fortunetelling, and ham acting to tell the bartender what he thought he wanted to hear. Two or three of the bar's other patrons, intrigued by the performance, came over to watch.

When Peter was finished, the delighted bartender gave him the beer and eggs.

"How about analyzing mine now?" one of the onlookers asked.

"Sure," said Peter. "For another beer and two more eggs."

The second reading was followed by a third; soon Peter had downed a total of three beers and six eggs. Others were still waiting in line. Since he was full, he decided to change his price. Moreover, he was afraid that if he drank any more beer, he would lose control and Johnny would take charge again. He began to charge $1 for each analysis. In a short while he had $40 in his pocket.

He left the bar finally and wandered away from the beach. A block or so away he found a cheap hotel and paid for four nights' lodging with his $40.

The next few days were happy ones for Peter. He spent each morning playing in the sand, watching the waves lap against the beach and the birds flying overhead. Each night he returned to the bar to tell fortunes in exchange for food and money. He quickly became an attraction in the area. People began seeking out the bar because they had heard of him. By the end of the four days he had accumulated another $200.

He decided he needed more clothes. He boarded the bus for town. But halfway there, he made the mistake of letting his mind drift—and suddenly he began experiencing the same dark, swirling depression that Dana had encountered several days earlier. For a moment his face went blank. Then his eyes narrowed, his face hardened, and he seemed to age several years. He was an animal, wary of his surroundings and ready to leap at any challenge. Johnny was back.

Two hundred dollars in his pocket meant only one thing

to Johnny—and that one thing wasn't new clothing. He began going from bar to bar. Before the night was over he even managed to pick a couple of barroom fights, getting kicked out of two places when the owners had finally had enough of his behavior.

The bar-hopping continued for two more days before his money was exhausted. Johnny, unlike Peter, had no intention of trying to work in order to finance his pleasures. He'd let one of the others do it for him. He lay down to take a short nap—and Peter took over again.

Dana might be ignorant about what happened during his periods of blackout, but Peter and Johnny knew all about one another. Peter was annoyed at the way Johnny had squandered his money and he was determined to earn more. He went to some of the downtown bars, hoping to analyze handwriting there as he had on the beach. But these bars contained a different type of customer. They thought Peter was queer and wanted nothing to do with him. He was thrown out of every place he entered.

He was saddened by the rejection. All he ever wanted to do was spread love and happiness. It upset him that he was not allowed to stay in the places where even Johnny, with all his crude behavior, had been accepted. Yet he knew he had to earn some more money. Then he remembered Dana's wallet, in the pants he had left in the department store. It had been filled with money.

He spent the next six hours locating the store where he had bought the clothes. He was in luck. The Lost and Found Department had discovered the wallet and he had no trouble reclaiming it. Inside was $235. Peter happily took the escalator down to the first floor and started for the door. But before he could reach it, Johnny took over again.

There was always action on Sunset Strip. Johnny took a cab there and spent the rest of the day drinking and trying to score with whatever women he could find. By the time he had had his fill of excitement he had barely enough money left to pay for a motel room. He staggered

to the unit the clerk had indicated and collapsed on the
bed.

And this time it was not Peter or even Dana who awoke,
but Phil—the fourth of my other personalities.

His head ached and his stomach was nauseated when he
first opened his eyes. He was not a drinking man himself
but he had experienced Johnny's hangovers before and
knew immediately what was wrong with him. He knew
also that he would have to fight to keep control; Johnny
and Peter must not be allowed to continue their activities.
If he could somehow get money enough to last him the
next couple of days, perhaps he would be able to return
home to Ann. She would be worried sick about Dana, although this wasn't the first time he had disappeared.

Phil remembered that Dana liked to carry a blank personal check in his wallet. He looked, and luckily it was
still there. Then he searched his pockets for loose change.
There was just $1.75—enough at least to buy some cheap
shaving gear at the drugstore a block away. He used the
rest room in a gas station to shave and make himself presentable, and then walked to the nearest branch of the
bank where Dana had his account. He cashed the check
for $100—an amount he knew Dana had on deposit.

Phil bought himself a half gallon of milk and began
drinking it on the way back to the motel. It helped ease
the effects of the hangover. He paid for one more night's
lodging and took a short nap. Then he went to a restaurant
for a steak dinner and plenty of coffee. He returned to his
room and slept another twelve hours.

When morning came he called the airport to reserve a
flight back home. He ate breakfast, took a cab to the airport, and called Ann before boarding his plane. He wanted
her to know that Dana would soon be home.

He remained in charge until he arrived at Dana's house.
Then without a struggle he vanished and Dana found himself sitting at his own kitchen table, facing his angry wife.

Dana didn't know how he had gotten home; he didn't
even know what day it was. His last memory was of being

in his car, just starting home from work. He didn't have the nerve to admit this to Ann, however. She wouldn't have understood. How could she? He didn't understand it himself. He would lie about this period of amnesia just as he had lied about all the others over the years. He knew she would give him one more chance.

But Dana's boss was not so forgiving. He fired Dana the next day.

CHAPTER 2

The mind of a multiple personality is like a rooming house in which two or more individuals coexist. When one personality is in charge, the others remain hidden in the inner recesses of the brain. Each acts independently of the others and is totally different from them in thoughts, attitudes, and even to some extent, in appearance.

There are actually two technical terms for the malady. One of them is *La Grande Hysteria*, the greatest hysteria. The other term is Hysteric Disassociation.

The word *hysteria* has a Greek origin, meaning "wandering uterus," and for centuries it was thought to apply solely to women. Even after extensive studies were begun on the phenomenon of the multiple personality in about the year 1919, most psychiatrists insisted that men did not suffer from it, only women. Today we know that approximately twenty percent of the recorded cases are male.

But the disorder itself is still shrouded in mystery, the subject of a good deal of controversy. Perhaps fifty percent of all psychiatrists deny that it even exists. In my own experience, two psychiatrists whom Dana consulted earlier in his life completely misdiagnosed it, because of their Freudian training and background. Freud himself, although he encountered it on several occasions, would never admit its existence.

I know it exists. I spent forty long years of my life suffering from it. Dana and those who loved him puzzled over it, trying to explain it away. Only when he finally encountered an understanding psychiatrist, Dr. Ralph Allison, who suggested the possibility that there might be several personalities living independently within his head, did most of what Dana had been going through make sense.

The key to understanding my situation, as Dr. Allison explained it, was that the personalities were totally independent, complete in themselves; they were not, as some people believe, simply separate facets of a single personality. Each one of these personalities had a different tolerance for alcohol, for example. Each of them looked different when he was in control of the body; each walked differently and had completely different postures. Since my cure, I have acquired first-hand knowledge of several other multiple personalities because I worked with them as part of my therapy. One of them actually suffered from severe allergies under one personality, but had no allergies whatever under another.

In my own case, I experienced an even more bizarre transformation. Before my sleeping personality, Henry, finally emerged, I had approximately 20/30 vision, and Dana was forced to wear the standard over-forty corrective lenses. After the fusion of my personalities, I went to have my eyes reexamined and discovered that I suddenly had the vision of a twenty-year-old. I threw my glasses away and haven't needed them since.

That suggests that the personality changes, when they occur, involve some physical transformations in addition to mental ones. Just how this is even possible, nobody yet seems to know.

Throughout most of my life, four different personalities

—Dana, Johnny, Peter, and Phil—alternated at taking control of my body. While Dana was undergoing treatment from Dr. Allison, a fifth alter-personality, named Jerry, suddenly emerged and made himself known for the first time. In several respects he was the most impressive and also the most puzzling of the five. He also remained behind after the fusion, when the other personalities had totally disappeared. Only recently has he begun to fade, and I suspect that he, too, will soon depart from my life.

But for most of my life there were just the four. Dana, the first of them, was studious, even something of an intellectual, with an emotional range that admitted of few extremes. He rarely laughed and even more rarely cried, and often was puzzled by the open displays of hatred, jealousy, even love that he witnessed in those around him. Yet his achievements in the field of business were truly impressive, especially considering the handicaps he was forced to work under whenever one of the other personalities suddenly emerged. My own career efforts, since the fusion, have not met nearly the same kind of success—leading me to believe that a normal, healthy emotional range can be more hindrance than help to a person trying to get ahead financially in the business world.

But Dana, while he was periodically successful, was also terribly lonely. Even as a child, whenever he succeeded in making friends with other children in the neighborhood, Johnny would suddenly take command and rapidly antagonize or frighten them. Johnny from the beginning was filled with rage, hate, and a barely contained violence that could erupt at any moment. Frequently he would beat up other boys and girls—and later grown men and women—whom he felt weren't responding to him the way he wanted. Naturally both the children and their parents blamed Dana whenever this occurred. As a result, Dana in childhood was considered "too rough" for others to associate with and had to learn to amuse himself.

If there was one thing that characterized Johnny, in addition to his total lack of compassion or morals, it was the enormous energy he possessed. Today I can only marvel at this energy; since the fusion, I am able to summon only a small fraction of it. His energy was such that it was almost a tangible thing; it often awed people and made them just a little frightened of him. It also gave him incredible strength. He was able, seemingly without effort, to physically beat up on other men half again his size, as well as to go for days on end without sleep or rest and to punish my body with alcohol and sex in a way that would have totally exhausted any other man.

In contrast to Johnny was Peter, who was as placid and loving as Johnny was explosive and filled with hate. Peter, whenever he took control, never hurt anyone. He was a poet at heart, able to express his passionate feelings toward life in ways that eventually earned him a certain amount of fame. Several of his poems were published. But he was still "different" enough from the other children in Dana's various neighborhoods that he was generally avoided, just as Johnny was. If someone referred to him as Dana he became indignant. "I'm Peter Pan," he'd tell them. "I come from Never—Never Land." If any of the other children tried to talk with him, he would discuss only poetry and a few other subjects that small boys and girls have little interest in.

Phil, over the years, appeared only rarely. He was, in the beginning at least, hardly a personality at all, but rather what Dr. Allison refers to as an "Ish"—an Inner Self Helper. Virtually every victim of multiple personality in time develops an Ish simply as a means of self-preservation—a separate personality whose sole function seems to be to prevent the other personalities from tearing the physical body apart and, therefore, ending their own existences. In Phil's case, he gradually began to assume some separate characteristics, and in time he became very much a personality in his own right. Toward the end, when he knew fusion was near, he actually expressed regret that he had been kept so busy bearing the burden of responsibility for the body they all inhabited that he had never had the opportunity to develop a real life of his own. He was, from the beginning, serious, seeming slightly older than the other personalities, with a maturity beyond his years. Emotionally his range was only slightly greater than Dana's.

To Dana, of course, the other personalities didn't exist. They knew of all his actions and conversations, but he didn't know of theirs. He had succeeded, after years of frustration and confusion, in blocking any knowledge of them from his mind.

At first he simply wondered whether people were lying when they told him about supposed actions of his own that he couldn't remember. Eventually he began to suspect that he might be mentally ill. He resisted telling anyone else about his suspicions, however, feeling that if it were known that he suffered from amnesia spells he might be locked away in an asylum. It was a fate he didn't think he could face. It was easier to deny that he had any problems —to lie and make up excuses for the things others said he did.

No one ever knew how little Dana was aware of many of the actions he was forced to take the blame for.

Adding to the problem was his own limited emotional range, and particularly his lack of sensitivity. He was never able to relate to others with the same illness and, through them, learn what it was he must do. He once even went to the movie *The Three Faces of Eve*, about a woman who suffered from multiple personality. Eve, in the movie, shared Dana's periods of amnesia and was shocked to find that people said she sometimes acted in ways that were foreign to her normal behavior. Yet Dana never related her problem to his own. She was, he thought, unique.

The greatest strain was on my wife, the woman Dana married more than twenty-two years ago. Ann had to live with a man who was totally devoted to her and his children one minute, then completely wild and irresponsible the next, often abandoning his job and his family for extended periods of drinking, gambling, and sleeping with a succes-

sion of prostitutes. Dana himself couldn't begin to express
whatever love he felt for her. Occasionally Peter took over
and wrote her poetry, but unfortunately Peter was often as
much of a problem as Johnny. He was scarcely seven years
old emotionally; and as likely to wander off to an amusement park as to go to Dana's job.

Ann shielded the children from knowing about the true
situation for as long as she could. The frequent absences,
she told them, were "business trips." The concern she felt
was never expressed openly. Only when the children were
older did they even suspect that all was not well, and then
Dana told them he had a drinking problem he was trying
to solve. It was not the truth, but it was an explanation
they could accept.

All this is over now. I have been effectively cured. When
I came home from my stay in the hospital I really was a
changed person—Henry, a complete man, and no longer
Dana or Johnny or any one of the others. Ann and everyone else noticed it immediately. My appearance had
changed, they said; my walk had altered, my eyes seemed
brighter, my speech was different. Best of all, I knew, was
the fact that I didn't have to fear any more amnesia spells,
any more of those periods when I would submerge again
and a totally different personality would suddenly appear,
to tear down or give away everything I had been working
so hard to build. I was one now, at last. Just myself. Me.

And only now, I feel, can I really begin to understand
the first forty-three years of my life. I am finally able to
piece together the unique memories of Dana, Johnny, Peter, and Phil—all living quite separate existences—and
make of them a unified whole.

That whole, as you will see, is not altogether pretty. I
have just awakened from a strange and frightening dream
that can only be termed, without fear of exaggeration, a
forty-year journey into the depths of hell.

CHAPTER **3**

In order to understand some of the pressures that beset me in my early years, and therefore to understand why my mind found such drastic means to cope with them, it would perhaps be best first to describe, briefly, my family's history—most especially the history of my father's side of the family. The Hawksworths have always been a little unusual.

Take my grandmother, for example. She was a high-spirited, dark-haired beauty whose family possessed both wealth and position as members of the British aristocracy. Her father was an attorney, or "barrister," as they are called in England. The king appointed him judge of New Zealand, a position similar to that of governor. The family lived in a large home, their every whim catered to by a staff of servants.

But grandmother wasn't satisfied with her life of luxury. She became restless for adventure, a fact that worried her father. He was afraid she might run off with some rough young man passing through the area. He decided to send her back to England where she could attend a finishing school that would provide her with a proper aristocratic education.

Her father was unable to leave New Zealand and escort her back to England at the time, but he knew of a middle-aged mining engineer whom he trusted completely. The man, Henry Hawksworth, was a staid, intelligent gentleman who could not refuse a request from the judge. He dropped whatever he was doing and went with my grandmother, returning to New Zealand as soon as he had seen her safely enrolled in the school.

Grandmother, however, was not enthusiastic about reading classical literature and learning which finger to raise when sipping a cup of tea. She accepted the school's discipline just three months, then fled, taking with her only what clothing she could easily carry. She had by then developed a fluency in languages and she was determined to use it to help her see the world.

She began traveling throughout Europe, spending time with first one man, then another, as the mood struck her. After traveling thousands of miles she joined a camp of gypsies living in Spain. The gypsies had been moving from community to community, telling fortunes, working the Tarot cards, doing whatever was necessary to earn their living. They were a closed group, but my grandmother's beauty—coupled, undoubtedly, with her willingness to bed down with the men—gave the leaders reason to allow her to travel with them. They soon taught her tea-leaf reading and the other tricks of their profession, treating her as though she had been born into their life.

In the meantime, word of my grandmother's running away from the school had reached New Zealand. The judge again summoned Henry Hawksworth and sent him back to England, with orders to track my grandmother down.

Hawksworth had a fairly easy time finding her. Grandmother had made enough friends wherever she went that her trail was not difficult to follow. He soon came upon the gypsy band and persuaded the young runaway to return to New Zealand once more.

Grandmother never talked about that voyage back home. There must have been a story or two there, however, because by the time the ship landed in New Zealand she and Hawksworth were engaged to be married. Her father gave them his blessing, despite the fact that she was still just eighteen years old and the mining engineer was already forty-four. He must have felt that the sober, hard-working Hawksworth would be a steadying influence on his headstrong daughter.

Less than a year after they were married their first daughter was born. A second child, also a girl, was born a year later. Hawksworth continued to be successful in his work.

Then, suddenly, something happened that was to change their lives radically. Several men came to Hawksworth with information about a fortune in pirate treasure they had learned about. They insisted they had proof of its existence—but reaching it, they said, would require careful excavation. They needed the skills of a mining engineer. Hawksworth decided immediately to join them, even though the work would require a long absence from his family.

What he had failed to realize was that Grandmother's faithfulness continued only so long as her husband was around. She enjoyed men too much to be without masculine companionship for any length of time. As soon as her husband left, she promptly began looking for someone to replace him in bed.

The man Grandmother finally settled upon, Reginald Farthingham, was a tall, handsome young soldier of fortune on leave from the Boer War. He shared Grandmother's "live-for-today" attitude, and the two of them were inseparable until it was time for him to return to his regiment.

When Hawksworth returned to his family after three years' absence, he was at first delighted to learn that a son had been born while he was away—until he discovered that the child was just a year old and could not possibly be his. To make matters worse, Grandmother had had the nerve to honor both her husband and her lover by naming the baby after both of them—Henry Reginald Farthingham Hawksworth.

Hawksworth was disgusted. He packed his belongings and left home, never seeing his family again.

Grandmother felt that children, especially a son, needed a strong masculine image around the house, so she quickly developed the habit of bringing first one "father," then another, into the family circle. Her life style was a little too unconventional for New Zealand, where her parents had been so prominent, so she moved to the nearby islands. But her wanderlust was still strong; she seldom spent more than a few months in any one place.

When her daughters were approaching adolescence she began to tire of the responsibility of raising them. She took the family to England and enrolled them in a private school. Only her son—my father—stayed with her.

She roamed England for a time, then moved to Canada and eventually made her way down the coast of the United States to California. During this period she never lived in any one spot for more than six months, and was still changing men as often as she changed homes.

Grandmother had her own peculiar moral code regarding her men. She didn't believe in living with someone without benefit of clergy. Each time she took up with someone new she had another wedding ceremony. A few times she even went to the trouble of getting a divorce. Of course, since she was still legally married to Hawksworth, none of the ceremonies was actually valid, but Grandmother was never one for technical details.

My father's unconventional upbringing was at the root of a good many of his problems—and ultimately of mine. My grandmother was extremely intelligent and he had inherited this from her. But the constant wandering had given him little opportunity to receive a formal education, so most of what he knew came from reading books. He had never had much formal training for anything, though he was able to learn fairly quickly when he began studying a particular subject.

Father also lacked a real father figure to whom he could relate. Most of the men who lived with Grandmother ignored him. A few abused him. Occasionally one of them might even try to get to know him. But none were around long enough for any meaningful relationship to evolve.

By the time my father was sixteen he could no longer stand life at home. He lied about his age and place of birth and joined the National Guard. There he found his first parent figures—the military officers—and began turning to them for the kind of guidance most boys turn to their fathers for.

He left the service at nineteen and held several brief jobs before discovering his real calling, as a door-to-door salesman for the Hoover vacuum cleaner company. He had a genuine talent for selling and quickly became one of the most successful employees the company had—this during the early years of the depression when no job, and especially no sales job, was easy.

My father married my mother after a whirlwind courtship in January, 1932, and I was born in March of the following year. The birth was extremely traumatic, and complications arose that nearly took both our lives. As it was, she was never able to have another baby.

My parents probably should not have had children at all. My mother knew little about raising a baby so she simply left me alone most of the time, taking care of my physical needs but little else.

My father was preoccupied with his career during my first year. He spent most of his time selling, and when he did come home he didn't want to be bothered with an infant. However, shortly after my first birthday his relationship to me changed. He became determined to make a man out of me. He seemed to feel that the lack of discipline in his own life had been a problem and that his son was going to be treated differently.

The particular method he chose by which to discipline

me remains etched in my memory, even though other
events of those first three years have grown somewhat
hazy. When I did something wrong he would first administer a violent spanking, then force me into an ice-cold
shower and hold me there until he felt I had "learned my
lesson."

The beatings weren't so bad. They hurt, but I learned to
adjust to them. It was the showers that terrified me. I was
little more than an infant when they began, helpless in the
power of this grown man. He would grip me tightly while
he turned on the shower and waited for the water to grow
cold. I would watch the harsh spray striking the floor of
the tub, my heart pounding as I twisted and squirmed in
an effort to escape. I would want to cry or scream, but I
usually managed to stifle that urge. Such behavior was not
manly. My father had told me so. Furthermore, I knew it
could result in further punishment.

When the water became properly chilled, my father
would grab me and lift me into the tub. The shock of the
icy spray would cause me to gasp and hold my breath, and
that, I quickly learned, only made things worse. I would
shake uncontrollably, curling my body into a ball in a des-
perate effort to gain some warmth. Even after I was finally out of the shower and dressed in warm clothing the
chill would linger.

I would do anything my father wanted me to do, anything at all, in order to avoid going into that icy torture
chamber again.

But my father was inconsistent. What pleased him one
time was cause for dragging me into the shower a few
days later. There was no way I could avoid his wrath, it
seemed—yet I desperately wanted to. Avoiding those showers became an absolute obsession with me. The fear of
them overwhelmed me—a terribly intense emotion for a
child who had only recently celebrated his first birthday.

In addition, my father moved our family to a new address every couple of months despite the fact that his job
was in a fixed location. As a result I never had any roots

and I never was able to get to know other children. I was a loner from the time I was an infant, lacking companionship of any kind.

Soon, like other lonely children, I began countering the emotional strain of not having real friends by inventing imaginary playmates who lived only in my head. The first of these, unfortunately, was Johnny. I would spend hours alone carrying on conversations with him. Shortly after my second birthday I was given a Charlie McCarthy doll and I pretended that Johnny lived inside it. I would hold the doll on my knee and make the mouth move whenever Johnny was supposed to be talking.

As the weeks passed, my imaginary playmate became increasingly real in my mind. I still dreaded the showers, but I began to think that perhaps I could avoid them if only I could convince my father that I, myself, wasn't always to blame for any wrongdoing. After all, I wasn't alone now—there was Johnny, too. What if Johnny was the one who did everything wrong? What if Johnny, not me, was at fault whenever anything bad occurred? Then my father would have to put Johnny into the ice-cold shower, wouldn't he?

I began blaming Johnny whenever my father became mad at me. If a dish had broken accidentally, I'd tell him Johnny did it. I tried to get him to see that I was good; Johnny was the one who was bad and should be punished.

My idea didn't work, of course. I still got punished. Sometimes I was punished twice—once for the offense itself and a second time for trying to accuse someone else of what I had done. Yet the idea lingered in my mind. I wanted desperately for Johnny to be the only one who was bad.

When I was three I created a new playmate. This was Peter; he formed in my mind shortly after I received a book about Peter Pan for my third birthday. The story, of course, is about a boy filled with nothing but goodness. He loves nature and can talk with flowers. He is 100 years old, yet he never grows up. He is tender and gentle yet remains all boy. He is able to express emotions I, too, had always felt, but which I had had to hide because they hadn't fit my father's concept of masculinity.

Just as Johnny was all bad in my mind by then, so Peter became all good. If anything went wrong, Johnny got the blame. But when I experienced feelings of love and joy, I let Peter express them. One day, for example, I was in a field and saw a beautiful flower in bloom. I wanted to share my discovery with my father, yet I realized that enjoying flowers was not an admirable thing to do in his eyes and might result in his punishing me. To avoid his disapproval I said to him, "Peter saw a pretty flower today." Then I described what Peter had seen, hoping he would think it was all right since it was Peter, and not me, who had had the experience.

Such attempts to suppress my real emotions in order to avoid my father's anger began to take their toll. No matter what I did, I felt I couldn't please him. Perhaps, I thought, there was something wrong with me—perhaps I was no good. I began to wonder why I should continue—an unusual emotion for a child scarcely three years old.

Then one night, shortly after I had gotten into my pajamas, I went into the living room where my father had just built a fire in the fireplace. There was no screen or grillwork covering over the fire, and a spark flew out and landed on my pajamas. Within moments they were in flames, and I was screaming in terror. My father rushed in, smothered the burning material, and put me to bed. Physically I had escaped unharmed, but I remained awake most of the night, worrying about the way I had behaved.

Johnny must have run into the fire, I reasoned. Having your clothes burned was a bad thing to do, and only Johnny did bad things.

But I had also screamed. I had cried and been afraid. My father had said that such things were bad, and a man didn't do them. I remembered the showers and began shivering with cold even though I was under warm covers. Eventually I fell asleep. The next morning, however, I was even more upset.

By the time I was ready for my afternoon nap I had worked myself into an extreme emotional state. I felt so guilty about the way I had expressed fear that I could not go on. I went to sleep, not realizing that it would be forty years before I would awaken again. Johnny and Peter, my imaginary playmates, were about to become quite real. They would share control of my body with Dana, a new personality whose emotions were limited. Dana would know neither true love nor anger. He would not be able to feel the fear and pain that had overwhelmed my young mind. I had become, quite suddenly, a multiple personality.

CHAPTER 4

Those early childhood years were difficult for Dana because Johnny and Peter were constantly experimenting to see just what they could do with the body. At first Dana knew what took place when they were in control, though he was helpless to stop them. He would explain to his parents and friends that Johnny, for example, had been in control when they thought they had seen him doing something bad. But everyone thought he was lying. They accused him of trying to blame someone else for his own misdeeds to avoid being punished for them. After a while he got into so much trouble over talking about Johnny and Peter that he tried to ignore them completely, and never mentioned them again. By the time he was about half way through elementary school he was successful in suppressing even an awareness of the other two.

One of Peter's earliest experiments occurred on a beautiful spring day. Dana was sitting in his back yard, gazing at a small pond filled with goldfish. As he watched them dart about the water he felt the all-too-familiar depression take hold. For a moment he thought he was falling into a darkened pit, then he lost consciousness and Peter took over.

Peter rose to his feet and walked to the fence. He stood on his toes, trying to see if anything was happening in his neighbor's yard, but the fence was too high for him to look over. He thought about walking around the house, but that would have required too much effort. "Wait a minute," he suddenly thought. "I can *fly* over there. I do it all the time in Never-Never Land."

Peter looked around the yard. "I'll need someplace high to jump from," he thought.

He decided on a cement gate attached to the side of the house. The gate was twelve feet high with a walk-way running through it, but the way it was situated, Peter was able to climb on top of it. From there, a smile on his face, he leaped into the air, confident that in a moment he would be flying over his neighbor's yard.

The "flight" lasted for only an instant—just long enough for Peter to fall crashing to the ground. He put out his hands to break his fall, but only succeeded in breaking an arm. The sudden, intense pain shocked and puzzled him. He didn't want to be in control of the body any longer. He had had enough adventure. He was happy to retreat back into obscurity and let Dana take command—and also take the pain from the injury.

Johnny was also experimenting, though he was interested not in imaginative flights, but in seeing just how much mischief he could commit without getting stopped. For example, there was a day in school when Dana heard the teacher suddenly calling his name. As he stood up, he glanced at the clock and discovered that it was 3:30. His last memory had been of coming back to the classroom from lunch. He had no idea what had taken place between that time and this.

"Henry Hawksworth, you're to report to the principal's office immediately," his teacher told him.

"Yes, Ma'am," said Dana, uncertain why the principal would want to see him.

Something must have happened earlier in the afternoon, he thought as he walked down the hall—but he couldn't remember what it was. He was still aware that Johnny and Peter sometimes took control of his body, but he had suppressed the knowledge of them enough so that he no longer knew just what they did when they were in charge.

Dana was shocked to see his mother sitting in the principal's office along with Mrs. Peskin, one of the teachers. His mother's face was angry.

Mrs. Peskin began speaking first. She had been coming up the steps, she said, when Dana had leaned over the railing above and spit at her. At first she had thought she must be mistaken, since she knew Dana as a quiet child. But then he had looked her in the eye and called her a "shit turd." There was no mistaking that. Before she could do anything, he had run back into his classroom. She had decided then to wait until the day was over to handle the matter.

"I didn't do anything like that," blurted out Dana, horrified at the story. "I never use bad words and I wouldn't call Mrs. Peskin something like that. It must have been Johnny. He was the one who was naughty."

But Dana was the one who received the punishment.

Johnny, in fact, was a constant source of trouble for Dana. He lived only for the pleasures of the flesh and the excitement of the moment. There was nothing good about him. He had neither conscience nor moral code. He could calmly torture animals and deliberately try to hurt others, caring not at all that they might be crippled or killed. Even when he was a child, murder was never far from his mind.

Several years earlier, when Dana was only five years old, Johnny's killer instinct first became evident. It happened shortly after the family had moved to a new neighborhood, where Dana did not know any of the other children on the street.

The year was 1938 and Nazi violence in Europe was a major source of conversation among adults. It was only natural that the children in the neighborhood made war their favorite game. They had sticks, which their imaginations changed into rifles. They held "military maneuvers" and practiced infiltration, running from tree to tree. The play frequently took place in the back yard of one of the more popular neighborhood boys—a back yard just on the other side of the fence from the back yard of Dana's house. Dana often sat alone on his side of that fence, listening to the happy chatter of strange children who would not let him join in their play.

One afternoon their indifference toward him changed to childish cruelty. They had been, as usual, merely running around, pointing their sticks at each other and shouting "Bang! Bang!" But after a while this activity had grown boring, and they had decided to bring out their "heavy artillery" and shell the enemy, who had become Dana. They gathered clumps of mud and arranged them in neat piles. When they had enough, they began lobbing the dirt balls over the fence in Dana's direction.

Dana approached this problem as he did everything else: He attempted to understand why the other children would want to throw things at him. He knew the missiles could hurt someone and he was certain the other boys knew it, too. Their cruelty became increasingly upsetting to him. And suddenly he felt an overwhelming depression come over him. A moment later Johnny was in control.

Johnny wasn't at all upset by the game the other children were playing; in fact he thought it was one he could turn to his own advantage. They were randomly throwing dirt over the fence, letting it land where it might in order to harass him. But Johnny had a far more calculating counterattack in mind. He went over to the small fish pond surrounded by rocks on one corner of the yard and picked up the heaviest rock he could handle.

Carefully he made his way to the fence and peered through a crack in the wood. He spotted the other children and walked in a crouch to a point directly opposite them. They were not even looking out for him, he noticed—obviously not expecting any retaliation from the mild-mannered Dana.

The fence was a low one, just tall enough to hide behind. It was no trouble for Johnny to take the rock, lift it high, and drop it over the top. He waited for the precise moment when one of the children was near so that the rock would fall directly onto his head.

Johnny laughed as he heard the sound of the rock striking the child's skull. The boy-fell to the ground, unconscious and bleeding, while the other children went screaming into the house.

The child was not seriously hurt, much to Johnny's disappointment. He had a concussion and several stitches were needed to close his head wound, but otherwise he was all right.

That evening the boy's father knocked at the door, his face flushed with anger. Naturally Johnny had long since disappeared, leaving Dana to face the consequences of the violent action. But his own father, to Dana's surprise, immediately began defending Johnny's behavior by yelling at the injured boy's parent. "Hell, it's your kid's own damn fault! None of this would have happened if your brat hadn't started it by throwing dirt clogs at my son," his father roared. "I'll be damned if I'm going to pay one cent for his injuries. Take me to court if you want! The judge will say the same thing—that my son was only defending himself."

In the end the boy's father angrily left our house and the neighborhood parents warned their children once more not to play with Dana because he was too rough.

A few years later, when Dana was in sixth grade, he and a friend began getting up at sunrise and meeting on the beach a few blocks from their homes. Their parents had given each of them a bow and arrow set for target shooting and they found the deserted beach an ideal place to practice. The tide was out early in the morning and the sand was covered with grunions. The two boys would shoot their arrows at the sea creatures, never hitting anything and never really wanting to hit anything, but enjoying themselves nevertheless.

But one morning it was Johnny, and not Dana, who met

the friend at sunrise. The other boy immediately detected the change, because Johnny was making wisecracks and his voice and walk were different, but he thought it was Dana simply joking with him. He did not realize how dangerous the situation was.

The two boys were shooting their arrows out toward the sea, seeing how far across the beach they could make them fly, when Johnny decided it would be interesting to murder Dana's friend. He put an arrow in his bow, took careful aim, and let it fly. The point struck the other boy just above the eye. The youth dropped, his face covered with blood.

Johnny came rushing up to see how badly he was injured. The arrow had not had adequate force behind it to penetrate the skull; nevertheless the boy was both shocked and in great pain. Johnny laughed with delight, then took off running down the beach, oblivious of the other boy's cries for help.

Dana suddenly found himself standing a half block from the beach, his bow and arrows in his hand and no memory of anything that had happened since the time he had gone to sleep the night before. He was unaware of his injured friend, of Johnny's action, or of how he had come to be standing where he was. It was only later that his friend told him what happened, though for some reason he never told anyone else about it. He told his parents only that he had had an accident. Fortunately he healed quickly after the doctor closed the wound with several stitches. Dana was still in elementary school when World War II began. His family was living along the California coast where, after the shock of Pearl Harbor, a Japanese attack always seemed imminent.

A Civil Defense program was prepared, and Dana's father became a block warden as well as a lieutenant in the Minutemen. The Minutemen were civilians who banded together to supplement the army in the event of attack. They built sandbag emplacements on the beach and mounted machine guns for use against anything hostile that might approach the area.

One afternoon Dana learned that several of the children were going over to the beach to play war games. He eagerly ran after them, hoping they would let him play with them. But as usual they ignored him.

Dana sat on the beach, well away from the other children, and watched them at play. He was upset by the rejection. After a few minutes he climbed to his feet and headed slowly back home. But suddenly he felt an overwhelming depression, his eyes glazed slightly, and his body seemed to slump. A moment later Johnny was in control.

"Those snotty jerks think they know how to play war," said Johnny, changing direction and heading for the home of one of the boys Dana had seen at the beach. He moved purposefully, his eyes narrow and hard. His body was tense as he walked and his fists clenched and unclenched at his sides.

The house was a block and a half away but Johnny reached it quickly. It belonged to a boy named Billy whose parents both worked during the day. The garage door was open, though, and that was what was important to Johnny. He walked up the drive, glanced about to see if anyone was watching, then slipped inside.

He moved quickly to the back of the garage, where he knew the family kept two BB-guns and a supply of BB's for target shooting. One of the guns was a pump type—the more times you pumped the lever that built up pressure in the chamber, the faster the BB would emerge when you pulled the trigger. If you pumped the lever enough times, as Johnny planned to do, the BB would have the force of a bullet for a short distance; it could even be used for hunting.

Johnny loaded the rifle, then pumped and pumped the lever until the pressure became too great for him to continue. He hurried down the drive and made his way toward the beach. He ran in a crouch, imitating a soldier working his way toward an enemy encampment. He was going to show those jerks what war games were all about!

As he neared the sandbags, he let out a wild shout and

began running toward the startled children playing in the sand. He raised the gun and fired at one of the boys. He paused for only a moment to pump the weapon, then fired again. One of the children felt a BB strike the side of his face, but fortunately he was far enough from the gun that it did not penetrate the skin.

Johnny moved closer, taking more careful aim. He wanted to hit someone in the face. If he couldn't get close enough to hurt them any other way, perhaps he could shoot out an eye.

The children were terrified. They ran about the sand-bags, taking shelter when Johnny fired, then jumping up and running once more whenever he paused to pump the gun. They knew they had to keep out of his range because it was obvious that he meant to hurt them.

The shooting seemed to go on forever. Actually it took only a few minutes for Johnny to empty the gun. When the BB's stopped flying the children stayed hidden awhile, then slowly they ventured out. Billy had recognized the gun Johnny was using and was as angry about the theft as he was frightened. He rushed at Johnny, determined to take the gun from him.

Johnny shifted the weapon in his hands, grabbing the barrel in both hands as he might a baseball bat. When Billy was close enough, he swung the weapon with all the force in him, striking the boy on the side of the head. Billy dropped to the ground, blood streaming onto the sand from a cut near his ear.

"I showed those snotty jerks," Johnny said to himself proudly as he ran across the beach. He reached the street and headed toward home, taking a route that went past Billy's house. When he neared the garage he threw the gun back into it, then continued home where he quickly submerged, leaving a bewildered Dana—whose last memory was of walking several blocks away.

Ten minutes later Dana learned what had happened. Billy's mother had contacted Dana's mother to tell her what Johnny had done. The woman was almost hysterical, even though Billy's injury was not as bad as Johnny might have hoped. He had to go to the doctor, and there were going to be medical bills that would have to be paid. But the wound wasn't serious. Billy eventually bragged about it, much like a returning soldier talking about his war wounds.

Still, Dana was thoroughly frightened. He didn't think he had done anything wrong, yet he couldn't remember what had happened during the spell. He knew he would have to take the blame, especially since the other children were so certain he was guilty. Moreover, he was frightened of the punishment his father would give him that evening.

But the shock of the violence was not so great as Dana's astonishment at his father's eventual reaction. The older man was actually pleased that his son would do something so manly. He warned him not to go around taking things that didn't belong to him, but he saw the incident as a whole as a boyish prank. The little speech both shocked and mortified Dana.

"But I didn't do those things," he told his father. "Those were bad things. I would never do anything like that. It must have been someone else."

As soon as the words were out his father became truly angry for the first time. "I don't care about the BB-gun incident," he said. "But I expect you to admit to it like a man. I won't have a liar for a son."

He grabbed the boy, pushed him roughly across his knee, and began beating him. The blows came harder and harder until Dana's body was sore and aching. Then he took Dana and carried him to the bathroom, turning on the shower so that only cold water was coming down. When it had chilled sufficiently, he thrust his son into the harsh spray.

Dana was terrified, but he didn't try to resist. He simply let the icy water wash over him, chilling him to the bone.

CHAPTER 5

My father caught the patriotic fever that struck the nation at the start of World War II and volunteered for the military. He had stomach ulcers, though, and was rejected, a fact that upset him greatly. Being a soldier fit his idea of proper manhood.

Later he heard about a job as a Naval Inspector—a civilian job that paid a Warrant Officer's salary. He decided that this might be an ideal position for him even though he had no knowledge of engineering, which the job involved. Fortunately he had a friend who was willing to teach him the basic skills he would need. My father had always had the ability to learn quickly any subject he wanted to master, and this was no exception. With his friend's tutoring, he was able to pass the test with marks more than high enough to get the job.

The Naval Inspector's position required him to go from plant to plant, inspecting materials coming off the production line. Each item being manufactured had to meet certain specifications set forth in the Navy Code. Those skills he had not learned before taking the test he soon acquired through training by the Navy.

The job meant more money, so once again he decided to move to another house.

During this period Dana became interested in chemistry. He had been given a small chemistry set but quickly mastered all the experiments it contained. The move to the new house enabled him to take over a section of the basement to build a more elaborate lab. With my father's connections in various manufacturing plants, he also was able to acquire expensive beakers, condensers, and other laboratory equipment. The home laboratory quickly became an extensive operation where Dana spent much of his free time.

The new job brought other family changes. My father became involved with people altogether different from those he had known as a salesman. His position as an inspector brought him into contact with high-ranking Naval officers, powerful heads of manufacturing plants, and other important figures. He was impressed with these contacts and enjoyed mingling with them socially.

Mother was a quiet person who seldom complained about anything. She kept her feelings to herself, accepting whatever my father did. However, she began to be more and more upset over his spending so much of his time away from home. Finally she began arguing with him. In my memories of those early years I seem to recall very few times when they weren't fighting. At night, hearing them argue, Dana would sneak downstairs and work in his chemistry lab, or just sit on the basement stairs, lost in his thoughts.

It soon became obvious, moreover, that my father was not being faithful to her. He began having an affair with a woman he worked with, and somehow my mother found out about it.

Apparently he convinced my mother he had gone astray only because she refused to spend time socializing with his friends. He convinced her that all would be well again if only she would go bar-hopping with him.

She had never touched alcohol until that time. Moreover, she was not an emotionally stable woman. It was not long before she was unable to control her drinking and was getting increasingly drunk.

The new job worked one improvement in Dana's relationship with his father, however. For years his father had ridiculed his intellectual interests. He had always thought that a "normal" boy should be concerned only about athletics and other physical activities. As a salesman, he had listened to his fellow workers talk about their children's successes in football, baseball, and track, but he had had little to say about his own son. Now that he had become a Naval Inspector this began to change.

The high-ranking officers and heads of manufacturing plants he now associated with were more impressed by intellectual achievements than the salesmen Dana's father had known. They seemed to respect the fact that Dana was so knowledgeable about science, and frequently they asked him about various aspects of chemistry and physics he was pursuing. His father could never understand why they praised these activities of his son, but he was pleased that men he respected seemed to approve.

Dana developed a few friends during this period, including a girl named Sally. She was intellectual by nature, sharing Dana's interest in science and Peter's interest in poetry. The only personality she did not like was Johnny, but she saw him so seldom that she generally chose to ignore him.

Sally was a year older than Dana; nevertheless they soon became quite close. She spent much of her time with him, often helping him with his chemistry experiments or just sitting and talking with him.

As the months went by, she began maturing physically, and soon became very aware of her own body—as well as Dana's. She began touching him and trying to get him to touch her in return. She wanted to kiss him when they met and when they parted, even though Dana was not yet old enough to share her desires.

What Sally did not realize was that Johnny was by now

emotionally ready for sex, even though Dana was not, and that her constant teasing was arousing his physical desires. Johnny decided that if Dana wouldn't respond to the girl, he would.

Late one night Dana's parents were having a noisier argument than usual. Both of them had had too much to drink and their voices carried through the house, keeping Dana awake. He left his room and made his way to the basement, sitting on the steps to think. It was quiet there and he no longer had to hear the drunken argument going on upstairs.

Dana was tired. Gradually he let his eyes close and his head sag forward on his chest. He felt a tremendous depression and a moment later he had lost consciousness.

Johnny stood up and started for the door. He was thinking about Sally and the way her small breasts were beginning to swell tantalizingly beneath her blouse. He knew what she wanted when she thrust them at Dana, trying to get the little bastard to feel her. But that chickenshit was too scared to try anything, even wth a golden opportunity like that. Tonight would be different.

Johnny walked across the street and around to the back of Sally's house. He knew where her bedroom was located on the ground floor. He stepped on tip-toe to look through her darkened window and saw that she was asleep.

"Sally," he said softly, tapping on the glass. "Wake up, Sally." He kept tapping, trying to awaken her without disturbing her parents.

She opened her eyes with a start, frightened by the sound at her window. She rolled from the bed, grabbed a robe, and pulled it on over her nightgown. Then she inched forward, cautiously, until she could make out who it was.

"Dana!" she exclaimed, moving forward more quickly. She was relieved that it was only her friend, though she was surprised at his being in her yard at that hour. It was too dark for her to see the narrowed eyes and hardened face that would have told her it was Johnny.

"Whatever do you want at this hour?" she asked. "Do your parents know you're out of the house?"

"I don't have any parents," said Johnny. "And that jerk Dana's parents are doing so much bitching at each other, they wouldn't hear the stupid house cave in."

Sally opened the window so she could see him more clearly. He sounded different, and she had never heard him use such language before. She looked at him closely. "What's wrong with you?"

He smiled at her, as though mocking her. "I've come over to fuck you," he said, putting his hands on the window ledge. "Open the window wider so I can climb in."

Shocked, she shut the window and locked it, staring at him as though he had suddenly gone insane.

"You no-good bitch! You feel up Dana but you run from somebody who knows how to handle you. I'm going to come in there and give you the fuck you've been begging for!" He bent down, picked up a rock and hurled it at the window. Sally leaped aside just in time, as the glass exploded into the room.

Her parents were awakened by the noise. The lights snapped on. Johnny turned and raced out of the yard and back across the street. As soon as he was inside Dana's house he submerged and left Dana standing there, puzzled about why he should be breathing so hard.

The incident totally destroyed Sally's friendship with Dana, a situation he could not understand. It wasn't until two years later that she was willing to tell him enough for him to piece together what had happened. But by then he had blocked out all knowledge of his other personalities; her story merely left him wondering how he could possibly have done something so incredible and then not even remember it.

Peter did not come out much during those elementary school years. The broken arm incident had upset him quite a bit.

When he did come out it was usually at night, after Dana had gone to sleep. He had developed a serious inter-

est in writing and used the time to work on poetry and
essays. Many was the morning that Dana would awaken
feeling completely exhausted, even though he knew he had
had at least eight hours' sleep—not realizing that for more
than half the night his body, at least, had been up and
around under the control of Peter. He was always surprised to find sheets of paper filled with writing scattered
about the living room. The pages were in a strange-looking
handwriting and were invariably signed with the letter
"P."

But it was still Johnny who caused the major problems.
There was one incident in particular. He once stole a
number of blank report cards from the school office. When
regular report cards were issued, he would approach other
children whose grades were not what they should have
been, offering to forge new cards for them in exchange for
a dollar. The new cards, of course, would show better
grades and would be far less likely to get the children into
trouble at home. The parents had to sign the report cards
as evidence that they had seen them. The signed fakes
were taken back to Johnny, who copied the parents' signa-
tures onto the original cards issued by the school.

Johnny made eleven dollars altering eleven report cards
before Dana got caught studying some of the blank cards
that had been hidden in one of his books. Naturally he had
no idea how the stolen blanks had gotten there, but he
couldn't protest because he had no explanation that would
prove his innocence.

Johnny, feeling extremely frustrated over his failure to
have sex with Sally, was anxious to find another partner.
His opportunity finally came when Dana was in the eighth
grade.

The girl's name was Jenny. She had once lived on the
same street as Dana. They both had been five years old at
the time; she had been the only child who would play with
him. Ironically, they had spent considerable time at childish sexual games in the backyard of his home while his

parents had been at work. Dana had been doing a lot of thinking about boys and girls and was curious about what made them different.

"Let's play doctor," he had said to Jenny.

"How do you do that?" she had asked.

"You'll take off all your clothes and I'll examine you. Then I'll take off my clothes and you can be the doctor."

The game had proved enjoyable, though neither of them had had any strong sexual interest at the time. They had played it a half dozen times that year, then gone on to activities that interested them more. A few months later Dana had left the neighborhood when his father decided they should move into yet another house.

Now it was May, and Dana's junior high softball team was playing against a team from the next district. A busload of pupils had arrived from the opposing team's school, and among them was Jenny. She had grown more mature with the years, but there was no mistaking her. Dana smiled broadly the moment he saw her. But that was the last thing he remembered. The depression came; Johnny was in control.

He was uncertain how to handle Jenny, even though he had no doubt what it was he wanted from her. He was aware of the games she and Dana had once played and he thought he might be able to persuade her to try a more adult "game"—if only he could get her alone.

He began talking with her, answering her questions about the intervening years. As they became engrossed in conversation, he gradually maneuvered her away from the noise and excitement of the ball game. Soon they were walking toward an old abandoned grocery store near the school. It had been sealed by the owner, but children had broken the lock on the back door so they would have a place to hide and smoke cigarettes. It was empty when the two of them walked inside.

Johnny was pleased that Jenny did not pull away in fright when he began touching her. He soon convinced her to let him expose her breasts, then to remove the rest of her clothing. Soon they were both naked on the floor and Johnny was having intercourse with her.

"Oh, Dana, that was the most beautiful experience I've ever had," said Jenny happily when it was over. She smiled at him and stroked his back. He had already started to get dressed. "I'm so glad I did it with you."

Johnny rose to his feet, a tight smile on his face. He looked down at her. "Don't give me that crap," he snarled. "An easy lay like you would go down with anyone." He started laughing, oblivious of the tears that immediately rushed to her eyes. She dressed herself, keeping her back turned to him, and ran sobbing from the store.

Johnny knew he had humiliated her, and he delighted in the knowledge. He took pleasure in the pain of others. It was several years, however, before Jenny could bring herself to even look at a boy again.

CHAPTER 6

Dana stood in the hallway, watching his mother ironing shirts in the kitchen. Her movements were stiff, as though she were fighting to maintain control of the iron. He wondered if she had been drinking. He couldn't see a shotglass from where he was standing, but he knew she sometimes took a drink or two even before he left for school.

His mother cursed as the iron sent a loose button flying to the floor. But as it struck the tile her intense expression suddenly relaxed. She smiled, then grinned; soon she was laughing wildly. He saw nothing funny about the incident, but his mother was suddenly doubled over in uncontrolled mirth, fighting to calm herself.

Minutes passed, as Dana wondered whether he should make his presence known. He started forward, then halted as he saw his mother's expression change again. She stopped laughing, took the iron in her hand, and tried to return to the shirts. Her face grew tight and she started to cry. She lowered the iron, buried her head against the ironing board, and sobbed.

Dana rushed into the room finally and put his arms around his mother. She seemed not even to notice him. He stood there helpless, uncertain about what he should do. His mother was growing increasingly puzzling to him.

The war had come to an end by that time and my father and my mother's brother had pooled their money to open an appliance store. My mother and her sister were also working at the business. Even Dana had to work there after school, sweeping up and waiting on customers.

Dana blamed his mother's radical shifts in mood on the drinking and her poor relationship with his father. But the truth was that she was becoming seriously mentally ill, a fact his father never seemed to notice. His life had become totally wrapped up in the store. He ignored her problems, just as he failed to keep track of how well Dana was doing in school. He could think only of how to achieve financial success.

As the months passed, Dana's mother became an increasingly heavy drinker. At first she avoided letting it interfere with her work at the store. She drank before the place opened and after she had completed her work day. Sometimes she drank at home, but more often she went to bars. Since his father left early for work and often didn't return until midnight, Dana was pretty much left to care for himself. He kept the hours that suited him best and used his generous allowance to buy most of his meals at a small restaurant near the appliance store.

His father's financial ambition, meanwhile, continued to grow. Soon he placed the family home on the market and bought a cheaper four-family house in a poorer neighborhood. He was there only for sleeping anyway—and he wanted the money for his business. But Dana's mother found the move emotionally unsettling.

The number and intensity of his parents' fights also increased to the point where the quiet times they shared were little more than temporary cease-fires. They both began looking elsewhere for the comfort they had once gotten from each other.

Dana was unaware of his mother's extramarital affairs until one day during the summer, between his last year in junior high and his first year of high school. He had taken a morning off from the store that day to go to the beach with a friend. When he returned home the telephone was ringing. His father was trying to locate his mother, who had not shown up for work.

Dana checked the house but she was not there. From past experience he knew she was probably out drinking. He began going from bar to bar throughout the neighborhood until he had covered the eight or nine spots closest to the store. A few of the bartenders said they had seen her, drinking with a soldier in uniform, but that the two of them had left together some time before.

Next he searched the bars in another area where he knew his mother had gone before. At the third place he found her.

The bar was a noisy firetrap with sawdust on the floor and country music blaring from oversized speakers along one wall. Most of the customers were low-income laborers drinking endless beers and an occasional boilermaker. His mother was in a booth, her eyes bleary, her face grinning happily. She was being fondled by a young soldier on leave from Fort Ord.

Dana was shocked. Had he been another child he might have cried, but such strong emotions were foreign to him. Instead he walked over to her, his face an expressionless mask.

"What are you doing here?" his mother gasped when she saw him.

"I've come to take you home." His voice was quiet, controlled.

"Look, kid," said the soldier, "you're not taking her home, I'm taking her home." He rose unsteadily to his feet, angrily grabbing Dana's arm.

"Leave him alone," said Dana's mother. "It's all right. He's my son." Then she turned to Dana. "I'm going home with this man. You run along now."

Dana wanted to express his anger at what was happening. He wanted to curse his mother for cheating on his father and to strike out at the soldier who was taking advantage of her. Instead he walked quietly home, feeling an emptiness unlike anything he had ever experienced before.

There was a liquor bottle in the kitchen. His parents kept it there for times when they didn't want to go out for a drink. Dana decided it was time to try some himself. He had never had a drink before, but he knew it could make a person forget his troubles and he wanted desperately to forget.

He took out the bottle and opened the cupboard where the shotglasses were kept. There were fourteen on the shelf. He took them all down, lined them side by side on the sink and filled every one to the brim.

The first drink was the worst. The liquid burned his throat like the fuse of a bomb set to explode as soon as it reached his stomach. A wave of nausea came over him and he began swallowing over and over again, trying to keep from being sick. But the one effect he wanted, the ability to forget, did not occur. After a moment he braced himself and reached for the second glass. It went down more easily.

Suddenly he felt depressed. He gripped the counter as his mind seemed to sink into a black emptiness. A moment later he was gone; Johnny had come out.

"So the chickenshit thinks he's a big man," thought Johnny. "Damn near pukes after a couple of shots. Hell, this stuff won't bother me."

Johnny drank four more glasses full in quick succession, feeling no discomfort from the liquor. Then he sat down, turned on the radio in front of him, and began drinking more slowly. Within two hours he had consumed all eight of the remaining shotglasses.

He didn't say a word when his mother and the soldier entered the house together and sat down on the couch. He listened to the sound of their laughter. The soldier was starting to undress her; he could tell it from the way they were talking. He walked quietly to the door and peered down the hall. The soldier was undoing his mother's blouse as they kissed.

"Who does that son of a bitch think he is?" thought Johnny. He went into his parents' bedroom, moving quietly so no one would hear him. Near the bed was his father's Smith and Wesson Police Special, bought during the war years and always kept loaded for home protection. Johnny took the gun from its holster and carried it to the living room.

"What the hell is that?" said the soldier, startled by the sound of someone coming down the hall.

"It's Dana. He's home!" cried Johnny's mother.

Johnny, holding the .38 revolver at his side, said steadily, "I don't know which one of you bastards I'm going to kill. Hell, I might even kill you both."

The soldier was terrified. "Look, kid, it's okay. I haven't done anything to your mother. I just brought her home and I was getting ready to go when you came in. Don't do anything foolish. I'm going right now."

"Yeah, why don't you get the hell out of here, because I think I figured out who I'm going to kill. I'm going to shoot my mother."

The soldier didn't have to be told twice—he fled. Johnny's mother began pleading with Johnny. She knew her son had been shocked to find her with the soldier; moreover she could tell by the way he looked that he had been drinking.

"You're nothing but a tramp," he snarled at her, "a cheap whore. You call yourself a mother to Dana but you're no damn mother. Dana might as well be an orphan as have a bitch like you around." He waved the gun menacingly. "You God-damned, no-good, two-faced. . . ."

His mother was terrified. She thought her son had gone crazy. She had never heard him swear before. She didn't know where he had learned such language and she couldn't understand why he used the name Dana as though it belonged to somebody else.

For a moment Johnny seemed to run out of things to say. He lowered the gun he was holding, then suddenly submerged, leaving Dana in control. Dana looked at his mother, then at the loaded revolver. His face went white; he dropped the gun and slumped to the floor. The alcohol that had hardly fazed Johnny had so overwhelmed Dana that he had passed out.

His mother, a rather small, frail woman, somehow found the strength to drag him into his bedroom and got him into bed. Then she went to her own room and immediately fell asleep. Neither she nor Dana ever mentioned the incident to Dana's father.

The summer following Dana's freshman year his parents' relationship deteriorated to the point where they could no longer live together. Some friends of theirs had a ranch in a rural area of California about 125 miles away. The ranch was small, but the couple also owned a feed store in town and their income was good. They had a guest house on the ranch and they offered to let my mother live there for a month. They told her she would have everything she needed, including privacy.

Dana accompanied her to the ranch and stayed there a few days, taking a short vacation of his own. At the end of the month she returned, having decided to try to reconcile with Dana's father. She hadn't had a drink while at the ranch and she seemed genuinely interested in getting herself together again. They kissed when Dana brought her home, and he felt hopeful that things might get better after all.

But within a week they were fighting again. Her drinking was, if anything, even worse than before, and she was spending more and more time away from home. Finally she decided to move back to the ranch permanently.

It would be the last time—except for brief, strained visits—that Dana would ever see his mother.

CHAPTER 7

As he entered his teen-age years, Dana's entire existence—like the existence of most boys growing up in the late 1940s—began to be dominated almost completely by the automobile. He lived for it. Remembering it now, I can only marvel that he, together with Johnny and Peter and Phil, didn't also die by it. They certainly had opportunity enough.

In those days it was possible to obtain a California driver's license at fourteen years of age. His father told Dana as soon as he earned his license he would give him a job handling deliveries after school. He would also buy him his own car and teach him how to drive it. Needless to say, when his March birthday finally rolled around Dana was far too excited to sleep.

His father had raced autos over the years, and once he had given Dana preliminary driver training, he took him out to a rural community for "proper" instruction.

"Start accelerating," his father said to Dana as they turned onto a long, deserted stretch of country road. "Go on. Put your foot to the floor."

The 1941 Buick picked up speed as Dana tensely steered in as straight a line as possible. The wheels kept slipping in the dirt, and the dust the tires kicked up filled the air. The speedometer needle hit 50, then 60. Dana was too nervous to keep watching it. The sensation of increasing speed both intrigued and frightened him.

"Stop!" shouted his father.

Dana began braking gently.

"Not that way, Dana! I want you to stop so fast that you put me through the windshield. Now get your speed up again and when I tell you to stop, tromp on that brake pedal with all the strength you've got!"

"This is insanity," thought Dana. But he accelerated again, thankful that no one else was on the road.

"Stop!" his father shouted. Again Dana braked cautiously.

"Dana, I don't think you'd deliberately disobey me by not stopping the way I told you to," his father said, his voice stern. "So I have to assume you're tired and you need a little air to clear your head. Get out of the car and run along beside it while I drive down the road a mile or two."

Dana didn't have to ask whether he was serious. The tone of voice his father used was the same one that had accompanied the cold showers. Dana got out and began running. When he was allowed back in the car, he accelerated on command, and when his father shouted for him to stop, he hit the brakes so hard the car went spinning.

After that the lesson went smoothly—at least as far as his father was concerned. Dana learned what amounted to high-performance driving. It was a skill useable only on a racetrack but his father didn't worry about that. He had very rigid standards for his son, and they included Dana's knowing how to drive a car.

For some reason Phil was the only one of my other personalities to learn driving that day. Phil mastered the high-performance skills at the same time Dana did, a fact that eventually would save all our lives. But Johnny and Peter failed to learn even the basics, though they were normally aware of what Dana was doing. When Johnny finally had a chance to drive, he picked up the skills as he went along, but never really mastered the techniques of handling a car at high speed.

Dana got his junior license the week following the training on the country road. Soon afterward his father presented him with a 1941 Oldsmobile. It had what was then called Hydromatic—an automatic transmission—and was more of a commuter car than anything else.

Suddenly Dana was popular in school, though he realized it was because he was the only freshman who had his own car. He quickly became everybody's chauffeur, never turning down a request from one of his classmates who wanted a ride somewhere.

Dana did have three true friends during this period —Ralph Potter, Larry Cardwell, and Jack Lesley. Jack came from a rather disreputable family. His father and older brother were both alcoholics and his mother did hard physical labor to support the family. Jack's brother had married a fifteen-year-old girl and the two of them were living with his parents. Jack was also a little wild, and really preferred Johnny to Dana. But other than those three, Dana was either ignored or used by his classmates.

Three weeks after Dana got the car, Johnny decided he wanted to learn how to use it. Having a set of wheels meant unlimited freedom to him. He quickly took control and for the next ten days practiced driving the California highways, sleeping in the car.

Dana finally awakened in northern California and managed to find his way back home. Oddly, his parents were rather calm about his absence. His mother's drinking problems and emotional illness had made her increasingly withdrawn from everything. But even his father limited his reaction to the terse comment, "I'm glad you decided to come home. I figured you would eventually. What the hell were you running from?" That was that. No lecture. No punishment. They just didn't seem to care.

When Dana turned fifteen the Olds broke down beyond

repair and his father replaced it with a 1941 Buick. This car contained a far more powerful engine than the Olds. It was just too tempting for Johnny. He had to see what it would do.

Dana arose from bed that April morning and started for the bathroom. As he put his hand on the door, the depression struck him. A moment later his face twisted into a half smile. It was Johnny who went inside to wash up and dress for school.

Johnny ignored Dana's favorite breakfast cereal in the kitchen. Instead he took out a liquor bottle and poured himself three quick shotglasses full. He drank them down so quickly he barely tasted them, but he liked the way they felt going down.

Johnny got into the car, started the motor, and drove over to pick up Larry Cardwell, Jack Lesley, and several others. "You sons-of-bitches think you've been driven to school before, but you've never had a ride like the one you're going to get now," he said, pushing the accelerator to the floor.

The tires squealed and the rear of the car fishtailed as it picked up speed. Soon he was going 80 miles an hour through the center of town, weaving in and out of traffic and slamming the kids in the front seat against the dashboard every time he was forced to hit the brakes. The only one who enjoyed the ride other than Johnny himself was Jack. He had never seen this aspect of Dana and felt a new warmth towards his friend.

The first period was English class. To hell with it, thought Johnny, I'm hungry. He left school and went to a nearby doughnut shop where he found a student he recognized from the junior class. The other boy was also cutting. They began to talk and he mentioned that he owned the 1932 Ford hot rod sitting outside the shop.

"My car will beat that junk heap of yours any day," said Johnny, knowing full well that Dana's car wasn't that powerful.

"You want to prove that?" said the other boy.

"Damned right I do," said Johnny. "You just name the time."

The race was scheduled for noon. Johnny wanted an audience, and he knew from the way Jack had acted that morning he'd be willing to go along as a passenger.

When the time arrived Johnny and Jack got into the Buick while the other boy got into his Ford. They drove to a waterfront area a few miles from the school. There was a dike along the waterway, and the winding road would make a perfect racetrack.

The cars started together. Johnny held his own as they went through the gears. The road curved and twisted about the countryside, forcing the drivers to keep their speed low; at that point they were still fairly evenly matched. However, its more powerful engine would give the hot rod a definite advantage once they reached the straightaway.

Johnny could see that he was going to get beat unless he did something drastic—and did it quickly—to cut the Ford's slight lead. As they went into a curve he swerved suddenly toward the other car, banging his car solidly against the Ford's rear bumper.

The other boy was not expecting the bump. He lost control of his car, spun out, and went off the side of the road. Johnny sped on until he crossed the finish line, then turned around and headed back toward school. He laughed as he passed the other vehicle resting in a ditch, not even bothering to stop and see whether the other boy might be hurt.

At school he began bragging about the race. He attended a couple of classes, taunting the teachers and starting some fights. At the end of the day several boys were waiting at the car but Johnny would have nothing to do with them. He and Jack drove across town at speeds approaching those he reached on the way to school that morning.

Jack's house was quiet when they arrived. The only person there was his fifteen-year-old sister-in-law, Miriam.

"You two want to go for a ride somewhere?" asked

Johnny. Both Jack and Miriam were enthusiastic. Jack liked this new side of his friend's personality, and Miriam was willing to do anything to escape the boredom of being alone in the house.

"I'm dry as hell," said Johnny. "Doesn't that wino old man of yours have some booze around here?"

They found a bottle Jack's brother hadn't consumed and each took a couple of swallows. Then they got into the car to drive to Sacramento, two hours away.

The car reached 100 miles an hour on the flatter stretches and balanced precariously on two wheels around several of the curves.

From Sacramento they drove through the countryside, still traveling at high speeds. Jack, who had climbed into the back seat with Miriam, was kissing her with increasing enthusiasm. His hand went underneath her blouse, loosening her bra. He unzipped her skirt and ran his hand down her leg. As Johnny pulled the car into a wooded area, he saw that Jack and his brother's wife were having intercourse.

When they were finished, Johnny said, "Listen, baby, you haven't been laid till you've been laid by me." He looked at Jack. "Get lost, you horny bastard. I'm going to screw her now."

Miriam liked all the masculine attention; she welcomed Johnny into the back seat. When he, too, was finished, the three of them drove back to Dana's house. It was midnight but nobody was home. They decided to have a few more drinks and one more round of sex before Miriam and Jack returned to their own home.

Dana was nauseated when he awakened the next day. He had a splitting headache and his tongue felt thick in his mouth. He thought he might have the flu, so he called Larry and told him he wouldn't be able to pick him up. He was going to stay at home until he felt better.

He went back to bed and slept until he heard the persistent knocking of Jack Lesley at the front door.

"That was one hell of a night we had, wasn't it?" asked

Jack, happily. "My brother sure picked a good lay when he married Miriam, didn't he?"

Dana forced a smile."Yeah, she sure was something." He didn't have the slightest idea what Jack was talking about.

But as Jack continued to talk about the previous day's adventure Dana became increasingly concerned. He had great respect for girls and felt that he could never do what Jack was describing—especially not with someone who was married. Yet he obviously had done *something*. If only he could remember. If only he didn't keep losing time.

Dana was also bothered by Jack's changed attitude toward him. Jack obviously preferred the wild person Dana must have been the night before. It upset him. He didn't think the things he was hearing were very admirable at all.

Jack, still recalling their recent adventures, told Dana about the car race and what Johnny had done to the other car. Dana knew the other driver would be waiting for him at school; he dreaded a confrontation. He decided to spend the following day in the city library reading books on science.

It was Monday before he had to face the other driver. Dana apologized to him for what had happened and offered to pay for the damage to the hot rod's front end. But the boy didn't want Dana's money; he wanted revenge. He insisted that they race again. Dana refused.

Weeks passed, and the boy kept pestering Dana at school. Dana was relieved to see summer vacation come around. He was embarrassed by what had apparently happened but had no intention of compounding the problem by agreeing to a rematch. He wouldn't race.

Then, that summer, the boy got Dana's home phone number and called to renew his demand for a race. Dana had thought the incident was forgotten; he was upset that the boy was so persistent. For two days he brooded about it, sleeping very little. The third day he fell into his bed, exhausted.

Johnny awoke, hopping mad. He left Dana's bedroom,

found the telephone book, and looked up the other boy's number. "Look, you son-of-a-bitch. You've been pestering that twirp Dana about a race. If you still think you're so damned good, I'll give you another chance to prove it. I can whip your ass any day."

He suggested a place in the west end of town for the race. It was a cross street, not nearly so safe as the country road, but traffic would be limited at that hour and Johnny didn't really care what happened. He was out for excitement no matter who got hurt.

The two cars lined up side by side. Johnny once more had Jack as a passenger in the Buick. They suddenly roared away together, crossing streets without slowing to see if anyone was coming. They covered the first block, then the second and the third, their speed increasing swiftly.

As they approached the fourth block Johnny suddenly saw another car approaching the intersection from his right, moving rapidly. The driver of that car and his passenger worked for the shipyards nearby, and he was hurrying home to retrieve his forgotten locker key, hoping it would not make him late for work.

It was already too late for Johnny to avoid colliding with him. He hit his brakes, slowing his own car to 80 just a fraction of a second before the crash.

Johnny's Buick, traveling a half car length ahead of the Ford, was struck on the right side. At that very moment Johnny blacked out and Phil took over. He knew how to handle the car, and he desperately wanted to save the body.

Somehow, Phil managed to move to the only section of the car where he could emerge unhurt. He also managed to save Jack's life. The front seat of the Buick was torn completely out by the impact of the collision. The frame was bent inward a foot and a half, jack-knifing the car exactly where Johnny had been sitting. Yet Phil apparently had grabbed Jack and shoved against him until the two of them had been squeezed together into the one corner not damaged by the impact. Fortunately the door latch had held. If the door had swung open, one or both of them would certainly have been killed falling out.

The people in the other cars weren't so fortunate. The boy Johnny had been racing had swerved to avoid the collision and struck a telephone pole. He was unconscious and bleeding badly. It would be a week before he was released from the hospital.

But the real tragedy was not discovered until rescue workers reached the third car. The driver was on the ground, moaning in agony. Several bones had been broken when he had bounced along the gravel after being thrown from the car.

The momentum of the crash had thrown the passenger of that third car under the wheel, snapping his back like a pretzel. His legs were completely paralyzed, and he spent the next several years in hospitals and nursing homes. Neither Johnny nor Dana ever learned the full extent of his injuries; however, from reports at the scene, he would probably be crippled for life.

Dana, after Phil had submerged, was bewildered at finding himself in the aftermath of an accident, though he felt neither shock nor fear. He had not been through the crash like the others, after all. He questioned Jack as the ambulance and police arrived, trying to learn what happened.

The police decided that everyone was equally at fault. All three cars, they felt, had been speeding recklessly. Tickets were issued to each driver, and that was the extent of the police concern.

There was a civil action, however. Dana's father was sued for damages by the passenger who had been so seriously injured. The man eventually received $11,000. It wasn't much for the years of pain and suffering, but Dana felt no remorse because he had not been involved. As for Johnny, he was glad the man had been so badly hurt. His stupid car had interrupted a race in which Johnny was leading.

In Dana's eyes, the worst part of the accident was his father's attitude. He was upset that a crash had occurred, but pleased, too, that his son had been engaging in boyish "pranks."

Dana's drag racing apparently fit his father's image of "proper" masculinity.

CHAPTER 8

Dana's high school years seemed to pass quickly, despite several other traumatic incidents that occurred then. First of all his parents, who had been growing apart for some time, realized they no longer cared for each other and decided to divorce. Dana's father had already taken up with an attractive redhead named Brenda, a woman of twenty-six, just eleven years older than Dana. And his mother had long ago given up on her own relationship with his father. They were living separate lives. The divorce would just make the reality official.

Dana had to appear in court during the proceedings. He told the judge he wanted to live with his father since his mother was permanently living at the ranch and he wanted to remain near his friends. His mother received a settlement that totaled $110,000, all of which was paid within the first year.

Soon afterward his father married Brenda and Dana began seeing his mother only during vacations and on an occasional weekend.

But the divorce was only the beginning of his problems. Dana's world really began to collapse the year he turned seventeen. High school had become a shambles for him by then because of the actions of Peter and Johnny. They had both begun taking control from time to time during the day. A teacher would begin lecturing Dana only to discover that she was actually talking to a seven-year-old child who thought he was Peter Pan. Or she would turn her back on Dana only to have one of Johnny's spitballs go whizzing past her ear.

Johnny had always cut school. During Dana's junior year, however, Peter also started leaving school before classes were over. Neither had any interest in what was being taught. Dana's grades dropped radically despite all his efforts to study hard.

His father finally was asked to come to school to discuss Dana with the school officials. The boy's behavior had become so erratic, he was told, that the principal was thinking of expelling him. They could only recommend that Dana see a doctor at once.

Dana was willing to try anything, including a psychiatrist. He didn't like periods when he couldn't account for his time, periods during which his friends said he acted like a different person.

His father wasn't about to spend money on psychiatrists, but he did send Dana to the family doctor. The doctor was a deeply religious man who used his beliefs as a crutch to hide his lack of medical knowledge. He would refuse to turn a patient over to a specialist even when he couldn't pinpoint the cause of the patient's suffering. Instead he would say that the patient's lack of religious faith was the reason for the problem. If someone couldn't be cured by the methods he was familiar with, the patient was obviously a sinner who needed to change his ways.

"You've turned away from God," the doctor told Dana. "You've been sinning. You must make a commitment to the Father of us all if you're ever going to stop acting so crazy. The devil's in you and you've got to drive him out!"

Dana said nothing. He didn't want to seem disrespectful by suggesting that there might be something really wrong with him.

"There are two missionaries living with me right now," the doctor continued. "They're good men who have found the *one true way*. I'm going to have them talk to you. They're the *only* ones who can cure you."

Dana doubted that the missionaries would be able to help him, but he had promised to follow the doctor's advice. Besides, he was curious about the religion the doctor professed so vehemently. As he expected, the missionaries proved to be fanatics who harangued him and told him he must either follow the life style they had chosen or he would go to Hell. Dana found their statements preposterous and refused to see them a second time.

When school let out in June of 1950, Dana's grades were barely high enough to pass him on to the senior class and he felt that he had to enroll in summer school to earn a few extra credits toward graduation. He decided to take courses he knew he could pass even with frequent blackout spells. He selected chemistry, because his home lab had given him an advanced knowledge of the subject, and typing because he had heard that the teacher didn't demand any work.

Then on June 25th, Dana received a double shock. First came the news over the radio that North Korean troops had invaded South Korea. War had not yet been declared, but reports indicated that the United States was considering a military involvement.

This news had barely had time to sink in before the Carson City, Nevada, sheriff called Dana's father and told him that a woman tentatively identified as his former wife had been killed in an auto accident. A head-on collision had taken several lives; the sheriff needed a family member to identify the body.

Dana's father wasn't about to take the trouble of flying all the way over to Carson City. He had his store to run, and he had stopped caring about Dana's mother years before. He telephoned Dana and asked him to come to the store to talk with him. It was only after Dana arrived that he told him what had happened.

Dana was horrified at his father's coldness. He was also shocked by the realization that he would never again hear his mother speak or watch her walk across the room. The emotions welling up inside him were more than he could handle. He certainly couldn't go to Carson City to identify his mother's badly battered corpse. He wanted to run screaming from the store. Instead the familiar depression struck him; he felt himself falling into the black pit. A moment later Phil appeared.

Phil was always in complete control of his emotions. He knew exactly what had to be done. He immediately made arrangements to fly from the airport nearest Carson City, where the sheriff had agreed to have a car meet him.

In Carson City a deputy drove Phil directly to the morgue, where the body was taken out for him to see. Half the face had been obliterated in the crash but he was able to make a positive identification. It was a sight that would have devastated Dana but Phil studied the woman coldly. He felt no emotions towards her. He was doing a task that had to be done.

According to the sheriff's report, the accident had occurred on a stretch of straight road between Carson City and Reno, Nevada. Both cars were found to have been in perfect mechanical condition and the weather had been ideal for driving.

Apparently the car in which Dana's mother had been a passenger suddenly swerved across the center line into the path of the oncoming vehicle. It had happened so quickly that there were no brake marks at all. However, Dana's mother's hand was found clutching the steering wheel in such a manner that it appeared she had caused the accident. Her boy friend had been doing the driving. Investigators reasoned that she may suddenly have decided to end it all; if so, she had done it in a way that cost four lives in addition to her own. Three nursing students in the oncoming car had also died.

Phil dug more deeply into the last few days of Dana's mother's life. She had been dating the driver, a carpenter, for several months, he learned. They had decided to get married and had stopped in Carson City to see his family before going on to Reno for the ceremony. They had been in good spirits when they left. But Phil realized that she might suddenly have had one of those radical mood shifts that had plagued her earlier, grabbed the wheel, and committed suicide.

Phil stayed in Carson City long enough to make arrangements for having the body shipped back to California. When he returned he met with Dana's mother's family to plan the funeral. Dana's aunts were interested only in dividing up her belongings and in trying to find out what had happened to the $110,000 she had received as a divorce settlement. It was a scene that would have been emotionally devastating for Dana, but Phil remained calm and in control. He never expressed whatever disgust he may have felt for the relatives.

The funeral was paid for by Dana's father, though Phil had to make all the arrangements. The family physician, a lay religious leader and friend of the dead woman, was asked to give the service.

Dana was bewildered when he finally resumed control. He found himself in the house, yet his last memory was of being in his father's store. He started for the kitchen to see by the calendar just how much time had passed, and as he went through the living room he noticed the register books for the funeral and realized that his mother had already been buried. The experience upset him even more than usual because it meant that he had completely missed an event of great importance to him. Yet he dared not tell anyone for fear they would think him insane.

By summer's end he was living in a frantic, topsy-turvy world. He had begun going steady with a girl named Cindy Myers who lived in a nearby town. He was also blacking out with ever-increasing frequency. When school started again, he often attended only one day out of three. Peter would go in his place one day and Johnny the next.

They angered the teachers, confused the other students, and kept Dana from being able to concentrate on his studies.

Cindy remained remarkably loyal despite the way she was treated when one of the other personalities decided to take her on a date. There was a night at a drive-in theater when Johnny was in control, for example. As soon as the first movie started, he moved over on the seat, took Cindy in his arms, and roughly tried to kiss her. He began stroking her breast, then started to undo her blouse. She pushed him away, shocked by his aggressiveness.

"Don't hold back, baby," said Johnny, again attempting to undress her. "You think you're too damn good for me?"

"You know I don't like it when you act like this, Dana. You said you wanted to see this show. Why don't we just watch it for a while?"

Johnny clenched his fist. He wanted to hit her, to force her to submit to his will. In later years he wouldn't hesitate to beat a girl until she submitted to his desires. But that night he thought of a better way to hurt her.

"All right, " he said, forcing a smile. "But I'm hungry. Why don't you go get us something from the refreshment stand?" He gave her some money and told her what he wanted.

Normally Cindy would have been upset by the request. Dana always had treated her with respect; in the past he had been the one to get the food. But she was glad for the chance to get away while he calmed himself. She stepped from the car, closed the door, and walked toward the stand.

As soon as she was out of sight, Johnny started the car's engine and drove out of the drive-in. "That fucking prude can walk home!" he laughed.

The dates with Peter were almost as bad for Cindy, though with him she was in no danger of abuse. The first night they were together he introduced himself as Peter Pan and informed her that Dana was not going to be coming on the date. He was extremely polite and wanted no part of kissing or holding her hand, even though such behavior would have been normal for Dana. He just wanted to talk about nature and poetry, subjects Dana never mentioned.

But despite all this, Cindy continued dating Dana and even fell in love with him. They talked about marriage after Dana graduated from high school. She had decided that she could tolerate Peter and Johnny so long as most of her time was spent with Dana.

In November that year, during Thanksgiving vacation, Phil came to the conclusion that Dana needed a change in his life. He knew that with Johnny and Peter taking control so frequently, there was little chance that Dana would be able to graduate from high school. He should drop out and join the Marines, Phil decided. It was something Dana would never have done on his own. He felt that war was purposeless and he was against the concept of the military. But Phil had decided to act in the way he thought best, and Dana really had nothing to say about it.

Phil went to the Marine recruiting station in Oakland. He filled out the necessary enlistment papers, and took those that required a parental signature to Dana's father's store.

Dana's father was delighted with Phil's decision. Not only did the Marines fit his picture of manliness, but the enlistment would also mean that there would be no further complaints from Dana's high school. The frequent conferences with the principal were a nuisance he could do without.

Phil stayed in control for a full week after he turned in the enlistment papers. There was a physical exam and a psychological test that had to be taken and he didn't want to risk one of the other personalities sabotaging them. When he told the teachers at school of his decision, they seemed pleased to be rid of him.

Dana awakened the day after the physical with no knowledge of what had happened the previous week. He was afraid he might have gotten in some kind of trouble and decided to stay home until he could find out.

His father and his new step-mother, Brenda, were not at home but they had hired a cleaning woman to take care of the place two days a week. She arrived while Dana was trying to piece things together and mentioned his enlistment in the Marines. He was shocked, although he pretended he knew all about it.

He rushed to his room and began going through his belongings. In a few minutes he had found the enlistment papers. Numbly, his mind whirling, he began searching for ways to cancel his enlistment. His induction was scheduled for January 28, a month and a half away. At least he had a little time!

Phil was aware of Dana's fears and was concerned that he might try to do something foolish to escape the service. He tried desperately to communicate with Dana, to tell him that the Marines would be able to control Johnny without hurting Dana. He wanted Dana to understand why he had signed him up.

Dana actually heard the strange voice inside his head and it frightened him badly. It was, to him, just further proof that there was something seriously wrong with his mind.

But as the days passed, Dana gradually came to accept Phil's point of view. With the war going on in Korea, he decided, joining the Marines might actually be a very patriotic thing to do. He would be drafted at eighteen anyway, and he was not doing well enough in school for graduation to be important.

By the end of December he was feeling fairly good about it, and even decided to hold a farewell party. His father and Brenda had planned to go to Las Vegas for New Year's Eve. That night seemed to be an ideal time to schedule it.

Dana took care of the initial planning and sending of invitations, but he was not going to attend. Johnny had no intention of letting him stay in control during any affair that included booze and broads. He emerged bright and early the morning of the party.

One of the guests was a younger boy named Gil Warton whom Dana had befriended while visiting his mother at the ranch. The two of them had liked each other, though Gil also appreciated Johnny's wildness. He and Johnny had occasionally visited prostitutes together in a nearby town.

Johnny had access to one of his father's Cadillacs and he promised Gil that he would pick him up. Jack Lesley accompanied him. On the way back, Johnny floored the Cadillac, powering it in excess of 100 miles an hour over a road that rose gradually to a height of 1,000 feet, then dropped back down in just two miles. As the Cadillac swept over the rise, Johnny saw that there was a police road block just below. He had no idea what it was there for, and no intention of letting himself be stopped. He kept his foot solidly on the gas.

The Cadillac swerved wildly around the long row of stopped cars, then slipped through a narrow opening in the road block itself. Johnny laughed as he saw the shock on the policemen's faces.

He hit the brakes once he had cleared the block, swung sharply into a residential section, then made his way to a quiet area where the police weren't likely to look. After remaining there for a half hour, he carefully made his way back to Dana's house. The police had even missed getting the license number so he never heard a word about the incident.

Dana had invited Cindy to be his date, but Johnny thought she was a stuck-up little bitch since she wouldn't go to bed with him. He couldn't keep her from coming, but he wasn't going to be bothered picking her up. He gave Jack the keys to the Cadillac and told him to bring her.

Cindy recognized Johnny the moment she walked in the door—not as a separate person, but as the one aspect of Dana's personality that she didn't care for. "If you're going to act that way tonight, I don't want to be here," she told him.

"You fuckin' bitch!" he said coldly. "I don't give a damn if you stay or go. But if you leave, I'm not giving you a ride home. You can damn well walk."

Cindy was furious. Yet she liked some of Dana's friends and decided she still might have a good time so long as she avoided Johnny. That wasn't hard to do. He ignored her, taking up with one of the single girls whom he eventually maneuvered into the bedroom. Afterward, he returned to the party in better spirits.

But he was drinking steadily and the beer began to affect his temper. He started arguing with Ralph Potter, one of Dana's best friends. He became increasingly abusive and suddenly Ralph, a member of the school boxing team, socked him in the jaw, sending him sprawling across the room.

Ralph thought the punch would sober Dana—not realizing just who his opponent was. Johnny rose to his feet, a half smile on his face, his eyes glaring. "You mother. . . ." he said, swinging wildly. The blow was more powerful than anything Ralph had ever experienced in the ring. He flew backwards, hit the front door and broke it open, sprawling heavily on the front porch.

Moments later, while walking through the living room, Johnny noticed that a girl named Gail had passed out in one corner from having had too much to drink. He immediately decided to have some fun. He kept an eye on her, and shortly before the party ended saw that she was beginning to stir slightly. He carefully stretched her out on the floor and put a pillow under her back so he could slide her panties off. Then he unhooked her bra and left her skirt hiked up on her legs. He threw the panties in the garbage can, hoping she would think she had been raped while she was lying there unconscious.

When he finished with her, he noticed one of the other guests trying to make a pass at the girl he had taken to bed earlier. He resented anybody moving in on what he considered his personal property. He grabbed the boy, pulled him into the yard, and beat him badly, breaking his nose, chipping a tooth, and bruising him all over his body. Then he dragged the boy into one of the bedrooms and left, locking the bedroom door.

Gail had regained consciousness by the time he returned. She was screaming and sobbing, on the verge of hysteria, convinced she had been raped. Her anguish delighted Johnny, who broke into laughter. Some of the other guests were also laughing, mocking the few who tried to convince the girl that nothing had actually happened.

The party ended at three in the morning. Cindy had already been gone for several hours, a fact Johnny hadn't even noticed. Gail and the boy Johnny had beaten were sent home in cabs—the girl still crying and the boy covered with dried blood.

It was close to noon when Johnny was awakened by a knock at the door. He had fallen asleep on the couch after everyone had gone home. As he sat up, he saw that the house was in shambles. There were broken beer bottles, cigarette stubs, plates with traces of food and other debris scattered around the room. The front door hung at an odd angle as a result of the first fight, and some of the furniture was still overturned.

Jack Lesley, Ralph Potter, and their girl friends were at the door when Johnny finally answered it. "We've come to help you clean up the place," they said.

"Hell," said Johnny, standing aside to let them in, "you sons-of-bitches drank my booze and ate my food. You can clean the damn place yourselves." He walked out of the house and drove off in the car.

The next two weeks went quickly. Dana made arrangements to leave school and spent some of his time with Cindy, who quickly forgave him for Johnny's behavior at the New Year's party. Then, in the middle of the month, his father and Brenda drove Dana to San Francisco, where he took the train to San Diego.

He didn't know it then, but his boyhood—as well as Johnny's and Peter's and Phil's—had just ended. His life would never be so carefree again. They were all about to join the U.S. Marines.

CHAPTER 9

Dana was not prepared for Marine Corps boot camp —though probably no one ever really is. While riding the train to San Diego, he imagined the training program as a sort of group bodybuilding course. The first day the new men might do ten push-ups to loosen up their muscles. The next day the push-ups might be increased to sets of twelve, and the day after to fifteen. In his mind's eye the Marine camp was a glorified health spa with information on weapons and warfare thrown in.

The reality was quite different. Training started that first day. Dana and the other recruits dropped to the ground and began doing push-ups. He had been physically active in high school, but by the time he reached the tenth push-up his face was flushed and sweat stood out on his forehead. Five more and his arms were beginning to ache. The muscle shakes began with the twentieth push-up, and when he reached twenty-five he knew he had had enough. His lungs burned, his head was tight, and his arms felt like jelly. He let himself collapse to the ground, breathing hard.

The blow caught him off guard. The top of the drill instructor's boot had smashed into his ribs with so much force that, for a moment, he thought a rib must be broken. He clutched at his side and turned his head to see what had prompted the blow.

"You think you're tired, Marine?" said the Drill Instrutor. "You're still conscious. Keep doing the push-ups!"

Dana forced himself back into position and began moving his body up . . . down . . . up . . . down . . .

Five more push-ups. Then ten. He let himself drop again, mentally congratulating himself for going beyond what he had thought was his absolute limit. Surely the Drill Instructor would be satisfied. It had taken a massive effort to accomplish those additional push-ups.

Another kick caught him in the same spot as the previous one. There was a violent jolt of pain as the boot thumped into the bruised area. Dana sucked in his breath and doubled over. This guy must be nuts, he thought. Vaguely he heard the Drill Instructor's voice telling him if he could move, he could still do push-ups.

Dana groaned, rolled into position, and started again. Up . . . down . . . His ears were ringing and his eyes were blinded by salty tears and sweat. Up . . . down . . . His lungs burned. His arms felt weak. Up . . . down . . . He became nauseated and dizzy. He thought for a minute he might faint. He became disoriented, but still he did those push-ups. Up . . . down . . . Finally it happened. There was a pit of blackness and he dropped to the ground unconscious. His nose hit the dirt but he felt nothing. The Drill Instructor came over and kicked him again. Once . . . Twice . . . But Dana did not respond. He was out cold.

Other joys of basic training awaited Dana. To accustom recruits to the rigors of battle, a dozen of them were told to put on gas masks and enter a quonset hut filled with a combination of mustard gas and tear gas. Once there, they had to remove their masks, sing the three verses of the Marine Corps Hymn, and put the masks on again. Dana's eyes burned and his throat ached for hours afterward.

They were subjected to a training exercise designed to show them just how much their bodies could stand when fighting in the desert. First their uniform pants legs were tied off so that nothing could fall through the leg openings. Then their pants were filled with sand—in the areas above their ankles first, then gradually up their legs and over their groins. When their pants were filled, the bottom part of their jackets were tied off so they, too, could be filled with sand. Strings went around each cuff to hold the sand in the sleeves. When their clothing was completely filled, they were ordered to stuff as much sand into their mouths as they could hold, and to crawl on their stomachs across a field without losing a single grain.

Even pleasure was made painful. If someone received a package of food from his family, everyone in the barracks was told to assemble. The food was dumped on the floor and the men stood at attention around it. When the Drill Instructor gave the order, all of them dropped to the floor and crammed as much food into their mouths as they could in ten seconds, swallowed it, and snapped back to attention. If any crumbs remained, the action was repeated.

Several times a day the recruits would gather in full uniform on the parade field. They would stand at attention while the Drill Instructor walked up and down the ranks, his swagger stick at his side. The stick—a short leather whip—was ever present and a basic part of training.

The Drill Instructor would walk slowly, looking at two or three men without saying a word. Then he would suddenly lash out with the stick, slashing at the face of one of the unsuspecting recruits.

"Did that hurt?" he would shout at his helpless victim.

The recruit would stand at attention, his cheek red from the blow, his eyes stinging from the tears he was fighting to contain. "No, Sir," the recruit would reply.

"Why didn't that hurt?"

"Because I'm a Marine, Sir."

Satisfied, the Drill Instructor would continue down the

line, repeating the blow every few feet. Victims were selected at random but every recruit felt the vicious sting of
the swagger stick several times during basic training. It
was a way of "building character."

Dana accepted the Marines the way he did everything
else. He hated the idea of war and the brutality of basic
training, but he suppressed his emotions and did whatever
was expected of him. The days were hell and the nights
were never long enough. He was allowed only four hours'
sleep—"whether you need it or not." He understood that
the Marines were trying to destroy individualism and
build a cohesive, machinelike fighting force that would
obey orders instantly. He didn't like the system, but he
had to admit that it was effective for the purpose for
which it was created.

He experienced the constant pain of overstrained
muscles that all the recruits endured, but the psychological pressures did not affect him the way they did some of
the others. His limited emotional range made it impossible
for him to get truly angry. He never became aroused by
the brutality of the Drill Instructor because such extreme
feelings were just not in him. Only Johnny could express
rage, and Johnny—at first anyway—had no interest in
basic training.

Peter also stayed suppressed. He was much too gentle to
want to be in charge of a body learning to become a fighting machine. The seemingly senseless violence would have
overwhelmed his tender mind.

Dana was able to tell himself that basic training would
not last forever. He had nine weeks to face when he arrived, but each day he survived brought him that much
closer to the end. He simply endured, congratulating himself as the weeks passed slowly.

Basic training had been going on for almost two weeks
when Johnny decided he was tired of being submerged.
Dana was on fire watch that night and it seemed the ideal
time to come out.

Fire watch in the Marines was just another form of recruit harassment. Normally they were allowed to go to bed at 12:30 and sleep until time to get up and report for morning exercises at 5:15. But the recruit assigned to fire watch was awakened at 3 A.M. and made to patrol the inside and outside of the barracks until the bugle sounded over the loudspeaker. Then he had to get the others up and tell them to report to the parade field. Officially it was a way to protect everyone from fire; in reality it was a way to deprive one recruit a day of two hours' sleep.

Dana felt the depression shortly after he had awakened everyone that morning. He was tired and unable to fight the feeling. In seconds the disciplined movement of Dana was replaced by the defiant swagger of Johnny. Neither Dana nor the Marines were ready for what happened next.

"So this is what that ass Phil got us into," thought Johnny, looking around the barracks. "No booze. No broads. What the hell kind of life is this, anyway?"

Johnny went to morning exercises with the other recruits. "I can do anything that chickenshit Dana can do, and I can do it better!" he said, taking pleasure in the way the body had developed during the past two weeks.

But Johnny lacked the dedication of a true Marine. He didn't make the maximum effort required and the Drill Instructor had to reprimand him several times.

Johnny began to seethe inwardly. "I could take that son-of-a-bitch down with one hand tied behind my back," he thought. "Smart-ass bastard gets a few stripes and he thinks he's some damned king." He slowed his pace, his face growing flushed as he watched the Drill Instructor out of the corner of his eye.

The D.I. was puzzled by the Marine he thought was Dana. He hadn't had any problems with him before but today the young man wasn't exerting himself. He came over and struck him with his swagger stick, yelling at him to get moving.

Johnny had not expected the blow. His face reddened and he began clenching and unclenching his fists.

From the exercise area Johnny and his squad went to

breakfast, where they were made to sit at attention and eat by numbers. This meant that the Drill Instructor would shout "One!" and everyone would put his spoon into the cereal. On "Two!" he would lift it to his mouth. On "Three!" he would put it into his mouth and on "Four!" he would swallow. It was a mass punishment for Johnny's actions during the exercise period.

After breakfast the squad members had to run back to the barracks, get their rifles, then fall out for morning drill. Johnny's squad was in the front line of Marines, all of whom held their rifles in the position known as "port arms." The Drill Instructor was in front of them, walking up and down, inspecting them. Periodically he would take the heel of his boot and smash it down on the toe of one of the recruits. "Does that hurt?" he would demand.

"No, Sir," the victim would reply.

"Why doesn't that hurt?"

"Because I'm a Marine, Sir."

The Drill Instructor reached Johnny. He eyed him coldly for a minute, then smashed his heel as hard as he could down on Johnny's toe.

Johnny never heard the Drill Instructor's question about whether the blow hurt. He had been slapped once by this mother, and he wasn't taking it a second time. He dropped his rifle, then slammed his fist against the Drill Instructor's jaw.

The D. I. was unconscious before he hit the ground.

There were two assistant Drill Instructors, one at each end of the column. They stared at the fallen Marine and then at Johnny. When they recovered from the shock, they rushed over to subdue Johnny.

Johnny looked down at the Drill Instructor, smiling. He didn't resist when the two assistants grabbed him, each man taking one arm. He merely turned to the one on his left and said, "I've had enough of this crap. You're all a bunch of bastards. You won't see me around here again."

Then the lopsided, sneering grin on his face vanished. His eyes closed, his knees buckled. Johnny was gone.

Dana opened his eyes, his body rigidly at attention. He saw the Drill Instructor on the ground in front of him and felt a rush of panic. He knew he was in some way responsible for the man being unconscious; the thought completely terrified him. To a Marine, the Drill Instructor is a god. He controls the recruit's every action. He represents the ultimate authority. It was inconceivable that a recruit would dare strike him.

The fact that Dana's last memories were of being on fire watch did not help his emotional state. He had thought after he joined the Marines that these periods of amnesia had vanished. Yet suddenly he had had one again; moreover it seemed that whatever had occurred during the blackout was going to get him into serious trouble.

The Drill Instructor regained consciousness as one of his assistants was still yelling at Dana. He got to his knees, feeling his jaw. His eyes looked a little unfocused as he stared ahead, trying to recover from the blow. He was a combat veteran who had felt his body could handle anything, but this quiet recruit who had never been any trouble before . . .

Dana's pulse was racing as he waited for something to happen. He expected to be beaten on the spot. Instead he was placed under arrest and led from the field under armed guard.

He was taken to his barracks and made to stand at attention against the wall with orders not to move throughout the day, though he was allowed to go to meals and to the bathroom.

When it came time for bed, he remained at attention. There would be no sleep for him.

The following morning, bleary-eyed, he was marched into the Captain's office for what amounted to a hearing. There he was read the charges against him, which, surprisingly, did not even mention the striking of the Drill Instructor. That crime had been so unusual and so shocking that no one seemed to want to admit that it had happened. Perhaps they were afraid that his defense would be that he had been struck first; the D.I. *had* stomped on Johnny's toe. Or perhaps they didn't want to admit that a still-raw recruit could deck a hardened D.I. with a single punch. Whatever the reason, the only charge was "disrespect for arms." His "crime" had been dropping his rifle, not the violence he had committed once his hands were free.

The punishment seemed straight out of a medieval kingdom in the dark ages. He was placed in what was known as a four-by-four-by-four—a cell four feet high, four feet wide, and four feet long. A man could neither sit up nor lie down. What's more, his only food was to be bread, water, and salt. This was to be his home and rations for the next three days. And as if this weren't enough, he would also have to spend an additional week in boot camp.

Dana felt a helpless frustration when the sentence was read to him. He knew that he had done nothing to warrant such a punishment; he had made every effort to be a good Marine. Yet he also knew that something had happened during the period of his memory blackout. Something had happened and he was being blamed for it. It was a paradox he could not fully comprehend.

The sides of the cells were solid, with bars running across their tops. There were sliding panels the guards could open to look inside and make certain the prisoners were all right. The cells themselves were inside a building to keep them from becoming extremely hot, but even this precaution did little to ease the discomfort of the men being punished.

There were no furnishings at all except for a brief period beginning at nine P.M., when the guards would toss in a pad to help the prisoners get comfortable enough to sleep. Each man could sleep from nine until four the next morning, assuming he could find a position that would permit it.

Dana spent the three days shifting his body, trying to reduce the aching he felt in his joints. Sometimes he would wedge himself at an odd angle so he could watch the guards without their being able to see him easily. Other times he would just sit as best he could, letting the seconds become minutes and the minutes become hours. He was bored and his joints ached, but he accepted everything without complaint.

After his release, he joined a new company that was a week behind his own in training, as was required by the sentence. He was determined this time to retain control and prove himself worthy of respect, and he managed it, too, despite an unusual amount of harassment from the Drill Instructor, who had been warned about what had happened earlier.

Eventually Dana graduated with honors. He was awarded the rank of Private First Class, which several in his company had been unable to achieve. He was finally a full Marine.

Dana's reward for surviving boot camp was a two-week leave; he used it to go home and see his friends. While there he met Ellen, a blind date arranged for him by the girl Jack Lesley was seeing at the time.

Ellen was unusual. She was only sixteen years old, but already she was one of the most beautiful girls Dana had ever seen. She had been in a convent school since the age of five, and Dana was the first date she had ever had.

Jack, Dana, and the two girls went boating together, drinking beer and generally having a good time. Dana was able to maintain control and thoroughly enjoyed himself. Although he was still spending most of his time with Cindy, he did jot down Ellen's address and telephone number, and promised to keep in touch with her after his leave was over.

Dana had another surprise at home. His father felt that if his son had to leave school and join the military, the least he could do would be to get into a part of it that would really make his family proud. So his father had pulled political strings to get Dana listed as a third alternate for the Naval Academy. Once he passed a competitive exam, he would be able to move up on the list; he might even be able to enter the Academy at once.

But before anything further could be done, Dana's two-

week leave ended and he was ordered to report to Camp
Pendleton and prepare for Korean combat duty. His advanced infantry training there went without incident, and
in June he was assigned to a troop ship that would take
him overseas.

When the troop ship reached Japan, Dana was given two
days to relax and see the sights. Then he reboarded the
ship and headed for Korea, a day's sailing away.

There he joined the other Marines in walking down the
ramp to disembark. Before his foot touched land, however,
he went into a depression, and submerged. He would not
resume consciousness again for several months. Phil had
taken his place.

Phil, as Dana's protector, simply did not think he could
handle the rigors of battle. Not only did he feel that Dana
would be unable to protect himself despite his basic training, but he also felt that Dana was weak enough to let the
other personalities take control in moments of great stress.
Such an untimely takeover could have disastrous results
—for all of them. Peter was so filled with love for all mankind that he might be unwilling to use his weapon to de-
fend himself against a North Korean attack. Johnny, on
the other hand, was impulsive and unpredictable. He usually didn't care what happened to himself or anyone
around him. He, too, might get everyone killed if he took
charge of the body, in a moment of great danger.

Phil actually welcomed the challenge of getting Dana
and the others through the Korean War alive. He liked
using the skills he had developed on his own and through
listening to the training Dana had received. He had already successfully saved everyone from several car
crashes; the war, after that, seemed to him to be just
another test of his abilities. Besides, it was he who had
enlisted in the Marines. The least he could do would be to
handle, personally, the consequences of that action.

That first day in Korea, Phil was attached to a mobile
rocket unit on the front line of combat. Some time later he
was with a group of Marines on patrol when they were
suddenly pinned down by a North Korean machine gun

nest. It was night. The only illumination came from the occasional bursts of gunfire on the trail ahead.

Phil and the other men fired into the darkness but hit no one. After several minutes the North Koreans decided to flush them out. One of them threw a phosphorous grenade whose flames both illuminated their position and killed two of the Marines.

Phil realized that he was in a life-or-death situation. The North Koreans had the upper hand, and unless he did something quickly he, Dana, and all the others would soon die, together with the others in his patrol. He took his rifle, dropped to his stomach, and began inching his way forward through the underbrush, moving quietly so as not to be detected. He crawled in a wide arc until he could hear the North Koreans moving about in the machine gun emplacement. Then he took careful aim and began firing rapidly. The North Korean soldiers were dead before they could react. It was an unusually risky action for Phil to take, and one for which, in time, he was awarded a Bronze Star.

Only a few weeks later Phil was suddenly notified that Dana's orders had been changed and he was to return to the United States. He was relieved that his mission was over and that he could finally surrender the body once more. Combat had tired him greatly; he felt he needed a chance to rest.

Dana, when he resumed control once more, was thoroughly confused. His last memory was of leaving his troop ship and walking down the ramp towards Korean soil. The ship had been rocking gently in the water, but that movement was different from what he was now experiencing. Now everything about him was vibrating faintly and the air was filled with the roar of powerful engines.

"I'm on a plane," thought Dana. He looked around and saw that he was one of a dozen passengers, the majority of whom were high-ranking Navy officers. The craft itself he recognized as one the Navy used for evacuations; he wondered exactly how he happened to be on it.

He was lying on a bunk on the plane. The seats had been

removed and the passengers provided with sleeping areas for the long flight.

"I've been shot!" thought Dana at last, checking his body for injuries. "That's why they've got me on this evacuation plane." He felt his head, his chest, and the rest of his body, but he could detect nothing out of the ordinary. He sat up, swung his feet over the side of the bunk, and stood up, still trying to determine what was happening.

Then he realized for the first time that he was in combat fatigues. At the end of his bunk was his M-2 rifle as well as the Smith and Wesson revolver he had been issued as a sidearm. He must be either going to or coming from a combat area; he just didn't know which.

There was a manila envelope sticking out of the mattress pad. Dana removed it and saw that it was from the Department of the Navy. It was addressed to him but he was certain that this was the first time he had seen it. Inside were orders, issued in late August, telling him to report to Bainbridge, Maryland, to prepare for the Naval Academy. He was to be there on September 10.

He must have passed the preliminary test in Oakland and been contacted in Korea. From his appearance he assumed he had been pulled out of the front lines so fast that he had not even had time to return his combat gear. So it must be early September, and he must be on his way back to the United States. He had served in the Korean War, yet had absolutely no knowledge of what had happened.

Later he learned he had scored the third highest of all those who had taken the test to enter the Naval Academy; that score had enabled him to become one of the principal appointments. He was proud of the achievement, because most of the men who went to the Academy were high school graduates. He was a drop-out.

He was also, it would soon turn out, due for a return to the life of total bewilderment he had been trying so hard to escape from. For while the war might be over for Dana's body, the other war, the *real* war, was still going on inside his head. That war, in fact, had hardly begun.

CHAPTER 10

At Bainbridge Dana was scheduled to begin a preparatory course meant to help those who had been away from the academic world get ready for the rigors of the Academy's college program. He was assigned a double room, together with a young man named Noel McManus.

Noel was also from California. His father was the publicity director for a major liquor company and extremely wealthy. Noel, himself, from boyhood had been brought into contact with leaders of business and government, a fact that had given him a sophistication Dana admired. The two of them became close friends almost from the start.

Peter was relieved by the sudden change in Dana's life. The idea of Dana's being in the military had been against his beliefs, but the Naval Academy was something else again. It was school, even if it was connected with the armed services. Peter would have a chance to take control and once more do what he enjoyed.

For the first few weeks Dana did well in his class work,

but soon Peter began taking over as soon as class sessions had ended for the day. Peter had no interest in the subjects Dana was studying and saw no reason to let Dana do his homework. He would much rather devote the time to his own work on his poetry and writing.

At first, Noel was shocked. He would watch in amazement as the quiet, unemotional Dana suddenly changed into a bubbly, childlike person with a high-pitched voice. Peter had an enthusiasm for life that was completely foreign to Dana. In time, Noel learned to differentiate between the two the moment he encountered either of them. Peter's bulging eyes, vibrant movements, and innocent face were easy to spot. Peter liked Noel, and the two of them had many evening talks on philosophy and other subjects that Dana never mentioned. But although Noel enjoyed the talks too, and seemed to genuinely like Dana, he realized that having two such strikingly different personalities was not natural. He suspected that there was something seriously wrong with Dana and suggested that he see a psychiatrist.

Dana was not surprised by the suggestion. He had known for years that something was wrong. Usually he tried to avoid facing the possibility that his spells of amnesia might be the result of a mental problem, but when someone as close to him as Noel suggested psychiatric help, he felt that it might be time to face it—and himself.

Noel advised Dana not to mention the personality changes right away. Instead, he should simply tell the psychiatrist about his problems in school. He had gone from being an almost straight-A student to one who was barely passing. It was Peter's fault, of course, but even Dana did not realize that at the time.

Dana did exactly as Noel had suggested. After their conversation, the psychiatrist concluded that Dana was only experiencing a delayed depression from his mother's death. He said he might also be suffering from mild battle fatigue. The grades were down, he said, because Dana had rushed into a school situation too soon after combat; that was why he was not coping any better.

Dana knew the doctor was wrong but he really didn't feel like discussing it further. He talked with Noel about it, though. He told him about his background and the fact that he had had blackouts all his life. He mentioned finding Peter's writings and being told by others how differently he acted during those periods of amnesia.

Noel also opened up about himself. He mentioned his fiancee, Jane Sargent, whose father was the governor of one of the northeastern states. And he talked about his childhood and the things that had bothered him over the years.

As the end of the session at the Preparation School approached, Dana was having second thoughts about going to the Naval Academy. One problem was Peter, who was preventing him from doing well—even though high grades in the Preparatory program were not a requirement for entering the Academy. That appointment was secure. However, he did feel his problem with grades now might be an indication that he wouldn't do well in the Academy itself.

He was also concerned about the amount of time he would have to devote to the service if he completed the Academy. Seven years was a long commitment, especially when the Navy was not really the kind of life he wanted. As a result, he put in a request to drop out of the Academy and let the next person in line have his appointment. He was transferred to Annapolis Naval Station for temporary duty until new duty orders could be arranged.

Noel and Dana remained friends even after he was transferred to Annapolis. Both had become closer to each other than they had ever been to anyone before, and they wanted to keep in contact.

That Christmas both Dana and Noel were able to obtain leave to return to California. They planned to get together, though their homes were more than 100 miles apart. However, when Dana called Noel after arriving home, he learned that tragedy had struck. Noel had fallen asleep while smoking in bed, letting the still-burning cigarette fall on the mattress. It smouldered, then burst into flames.

The poisoned fumes that resulted had taken Noel's life.

Dana felt a tremendous emptiness when he learned of his friend's death. He wanted to cry or in some way express some deep feeling about what had happened. But he couldn't; his range of emotions was too narrow. He was saddened, but that was all. Noel had been the closest friend he had ever had. Yet much as he wanted to, he simply couldn't mourn his passing so deeply that he could be moved to tears.

Noel's family wanted Dana to act as a pall bearer but he wanted no part of the funeral. Perhaps, had he been able to feel a greater range of emotions, he might at least have gone to see the family. But he felt that with his friend dead, any involvement with the parents would be pointless.

Two weeks later Dana received a telephone call from Jane Sargent, Noel's former fiancee. Apparently Noel had told her about his friendship with Dana. Now Jane suggested that if the two of them could meet, they might be able to talk about Noel and in that way ease the pain of their loss.

Dana didn't want to get involved with Jane, but felt that he owed it to Noel to give her what comfort he could. They agreed to meet after Dana returned to his base in a few days.

The first weekend he was back he was granted a forty-eight-hour pass, and he and Jane met in a small Washington restaurant they both knew. The conversation centered on Noel and the last talks he had had with Dana.

Dana returned to the base thinking that he would never see Jane again. He had found her attractive but felt that they would now go their separate ways. To his surprise, however, she wrote to him several days later and asked if he would come to her college to see her.

The relationship with Jane changed during that second weekend. Dana couldn't tell if she had turned to him as a substitute for Noel or if she genuinely was becoming interested in him, but whichever was the case, their talk soon turned to themselves, their plans for the future, and all the other things couples discuss when becoming serious about each other. They began seeing each other as often as possible.

After several months Dana was transferred to the Marine base in North Carolina. He was given two weeks' leave before he had to report for duty and he used the time to go home. While there, he dated his high school sweetheart, Cindy, but found himself cooling on their relationship. He told her finally that he was dating others and was not certain he still wanted to marry her. To underscore the point, he asked Ellen for a date and she accepted.

What Ellen didn't realize was that Dana was not the person who would pick her up.

Johnny had been interested in Ellen, despite the fact that she was still very young, from the moment Dana met her. He had never seen anyone so pretty and he liked the idea of her having spent so many years in a convent school. He saw her as ripe for the taking and he intended to be the one to take her—regardless of what she, or Dana, might want.

Dana had been given permission to use his father's Cadillac on the date and Johnny saw no reason to leave it behind. He drove to Ellen's house, honked the horn, and waited for her to appear. She was going to spend the evening with a real man, so the least she could do was come running. That wasn't the way that chickenshit Dana would do things, but there were a lot of things Dana wouldn't do that Johnny had planned for the evening.

He floored the accelerator as soon as Ellen climbed into the car. The Cadillac screeched from the curb and bounded down the street. They reached the corner and Johnny turned sharply, not bothering to brake. The car swung wide, two wheels rising off the ground. He was going to show her what a Cadillac could do with someone behind the wheel who knew how to put it through its paces.

Ellen was frightened. Her face was pale and her hands clutched the edge of the seat so tightly that her knuckles turned white. She had thought Dana was much quieter than this. She wondered what had happened to him in the Marines.

The car raced into the countryside and up into the mountains. There was a small restaurant and bar Dana had been to once, and Johnny thought it was the ideal place to take Ellen. They had a sandwich there and Johnny encouraged her to drink beer. She nursed the first, but drank the second a little faster. He bought her a third; soon she was in a more receptive mood.

Finally he took her back to the car, both of them light-headed from the beer. He drove up the road a little farther, turning off into a heavily wooded area. He moved close beside her, put his arm around her, and kissed her. When he felt her respond to his kissing he fondled her breast through her blouse, then reached for the buttons.

"Don't, Dana," she said softly, taking his hand.

"Don't, Dana," he mocked. That chickenshit wouldn't have the nerve, he thought.

He jerked his hand free of hers and began pulling open the blouse. When she protested he muffled her cries by kissing her hard, hurting her lips. He forced her arm back to keep her from interfering.

Ellen struggled frantically as Johnny unhooked her bra and began pulling it off. Suddenly he slapped her hard, across the face. "Don't act like that, you bitch. You're going to have it with a real man and you're going to love it."

"Please, Dana, I'm not like that. Please. Don't do this." Her voice was trembling and she seemed near tears. She pushed against him, trying to get free, but he slapped her again.

"Don't act innocent with me, you bitch. You've been ask-.ing for this from the moment I saw you." She was naked to the waist and he was undoing her skirt. He held her wrists with one hand and kissed her again hard.

He removed her skirt, running his hand between her legs. He kissed her again and realized suddenly that she had stopped struggling. When he released her hands she

actually reached over and began loosening his belt. Her
face became flushed as she tore at his clothing. In a few
moments they were having intercourse. What had started
as a rape had sexually excited the girl; she responded with
a passion at least as strong as his own. He was delighted.
He liked the idea of a girl who could be turned on by his
violence.

It wasn't until much later that Johnny, through Dana,
would learn the reasons behind Ellen's surprising reaction.
It was true that she had attended a convent school all her
life, but she had not been placed in the school because of
the strict moral code of her parents. In fact she did not
even know who her father was, and it was unlikely that he
had ever been married to her mother.

For Ellen's mother, it turned out, was a successful independent businesswoman in the world's oldest profession.
She was a top strip-tease dancer and one of the highest-
priced prostitutes in San Francisco. She had placed her
daughter in the convent school to give her a good education and the kind of discipline she had been unable to provide because of her unusual working hours. But the
mother had also passed along to Ellen her "street sense"
about men and sex, thus giving her not only sophistication
and beauty, but also an understanding of men that made
her quite exciting.

Ellen decided that she was in love with Dana after her
experience with Johnny. She realized that Dana was not
always as aggressive as he had been that day, but she
liked his violent side enough to put up with his more reserved moods, too. She began calling him at home, often
two or three times a day. Dana couldn't understand the
reason for such attention, and he couldn't remember the
date she kept discussing either.

He decided to go out with Ellen one more time before
returning to base, and that time Johnny, for some reason,
did not take over. The date proved to be a major disappointment for Ellen. Dana had only limited interest in
girls and no desire at all to have sexual relations with a

girl he hardly knew. He drove her into the hills overlooking the city, put his arm around her, and kissed her. But
he ignored her efforts to get him to go further. By the time
he took her home, she was both frustrated and puzzled by
his restraint. It was a most unsatisfactory evening for both
of them.

When Dana's leave came to an end he reported to Camp
Lejeune, where he was assigned the position of forward
observer for an artillery company. He accepted the situation as he accepted everything else that had happened to
him, expressing no regret even though the base was considered by the Marines to be the worst in the country. Camp
Lejeune was totally isolated. The passes issued to Marines
stationed there were for one day longer than passes issued
by any other Marine base, so that the men there would
have time to travel all the way to "civilization."

When Dana's first four-day pass came through, he contacted Jane and suggested they meet in Baltimore. She
had a number of friends there with whom she could stay
and he would take a hotel room. The hotel room proved
unnecessary, however. Jane replied that she had arranged
for both of them to stay with the family of a socially prominent friend of hers from school.

On his second night there Dana took Jane to dinner and
a floor show at one of the Baltimore night spots. As they
sat drinking in the lounge following the show, Johnny decided that it was only right for him to enjoy Dana's leave,
too.

Jane was shocked as she watched the sudden transformation take place. Dana had just taken a sip from his second drink when his eyes glazed over. The lids narrowed
and his face stiffened. His muscles tensed and he brought
the drink back to his mouth, swallowing it all at once instead of slowly nursing it the way Dana normally did. He
ordered another drink, finished it before the cocktail waitress could go, then ordered one more. "You're not a bad-
looking broad," he said, looking Jane over critically. He
added matter-of-factly, "I don't know why that chickenshit
never laid you."

The sudden change in him completely amazed her. She would have sworn she was seeing a different man from the one who had brought her to the club. She was frightened, though she wasn't certain just why.

Johnny kept drinking steadily, his conversation growing increasingly lurid and abusive.

"I . . . I think we'd better be getting back," said Jane nervously. She had never heard him talk like that and was anxious to end the evening.

Johnny got in the car and pressed the accelerator to the floor. The car shot from the parking lot, fishtailing on the road until the tires gained a little traction. He drove as fast as he could, spinning wildly around corners and narrowly missing parked cars. Jane braced herself against the dash and prayed they would make it back safely.

There was a large circular drive in front of the house in which they were both staying. Although some lights had been left on inside, the drive area was dark when Johnny pulled the car to the door. He took Jane in his arms and tried to have sex with her as he had with Ellen several weeks before. Jane was not the same kind of girl, however. She pushed him back, opened her door, and stalked angrily into the house.

Johnny laughed at the fleeing figure, then started the car's engine and drove away in a spray of loose gravel. At nine the next morning, Lisa Mason, the friend with whom they were staying, found Dana asleep in the back seat of the car parked in the driveway. She shook him awake and asked him why he hadn't gone in to bed. He didn't know.

Jane was rather cold toward Dana that day. The following morning he had to return to base and she agreed to drive him to the bus station. It was then that he finally learned what had taken place the night before.

"I'm sorry about what happened, " Dana told her. He was becoming skilled at making excuses for behavior he couldn't explain and didn't remember. "When I was in Korea I developed a personality problem. It has something to do with combat pressures, I guess. I'm trying to get over it, but when I drink too much it sometimes comes out."

The explanation seemed to satisfy Jane, in part because she wanted it to satisfy her. She didn't want to lose Dana because of one unpleasant experience. She apologized for staying angry at him so long.

During the next couple of months Dana was bewildered to find himself the object of love letters from three different girls. Cindy continued to write despite his efforts to cool their high school romance, and Jane also sent passionate notes. In addition, Ellen, the seventeen-year-old girl Johnny had seduced, sent him a Polaroid picture of herself taken in the nude. She told him her body was his if he would have her. She wanted to run away from home and come live in North Carolina, just off his base. She would take an apartment and find a job, she said, just to be near him.

Dana was surprised by Ellen's letter. He enjoyed looking at the photograph but the idea of having her live nearby to be with him didn't appeal to him at all. He felt that she was too young, that she had no idea what she might be getting herself into. He certainly had no interest in marrying the girl, and anything less than marriage went against his moral code. He also was concerned that she might really be in love with the kind of person he became only during some of his amnesia periods.

Ellen was not yet of legal age, and Dana decided to use that fact to tell her not to come. He explained that because of her age she could get them both in trouble. He tried to sound like a big brother, hoping to be cool enough to get the message across without sounding cruel.

Meanwhile, Jane's summer vacation was scheduled to begin at the end of June and she asked Dana if he could go home with her. She said she would pick him up and together they could drive to the governor's mansion in the state where she lived. He was able to get a pass and looked forward eagerly to the trip.

The governor's mansion was overwhelming. Its grounds consisted of several acres, all beautifully landscaped, near the heart of the state capital. There were more than twenty rooms, a garage large enough for six cars, and a staff of servants to handle everything from maintenance to the preparation of the meals. Most of the cost of the mansion was met by the taxpayers; the rest was paid for from the governor's considerable personal wealth.

On his first day there Dana met the governor, an imposing man who immediately set him at ease, and the governor's wife, Jane's mother, who was quiet but friendly. Neither Johnny nor Peter had any interest in seeing the place at that point, so Dana remained in control. He spent the evening alone with Jane, then was shown to his room at eleven when they both were getting tired.

The mansion's guest room was impressive indeed. It was behind the garage to give it a measure of privacy, though it was reached through a hall in the house. But its size was awesome. It had a bedroom, sitting room, kitchen, and bath. It was as large as many apartments, and it completely overwhelmed Dana.

He had been asleep for two or three hours that first night when he felt someone shaking him gently. A night-light had been turned on by the door and, as his eyes focused, he was able to see Jane standing beside his bed. She smiled. "You're a sound sleeper, Dana," she said.

She was wearing red "baby doll" pajamas and her soft brown hair, normally tied up in a bun, cascaded down her back and over one shoulder. Her glasses were off and what little make-up she had on enhanced her seductiveness.

Her presence both shocked him and stimulated him sexually. Her seductiveness delighted him, but her being there seemed as out of character to him as Johnny had seemed out of character to her. "What are you doing here?" he asked.

"I've been thinking about you ever since we said good-night," she said, pushing back the covers as she sat on the bed. "I want to prove to you that I love you." She swung her feet off the floor and stretched out on the bed close to him. Gently, her hand touched his face.

"You don't have to prove your love," said Dana uneasily.

"I've never wanted you to do anything with me to prove how you feel. I mean. . . . " Her hand went down his side, stroking his leg.

"You say that, but I know differently," she said, kissing him. "The last few times we were together you changed at the end of the evening. You wanted to have sex with me but I refused. You acted like a wild man and it upset me." She slipped off her pajama top and pressed against him.

"But . . . Jane, I told you about my behavior problem," Dana said, gulping noisily. "I wasn't myself when I made those passes at you. You did the right thing in refusing me."

"You're sweet to say that, Dana. And I want you to know that the only man I've ever been to bed with was Noel. I loved him and felt no shame in what we did. With you I also feel no shame. You want me and I want you. There's no reason you shouldn't have me, no matter what happened on our other dates."

Dana may have had a limited emotional range but he was far from being totally insensitive. The fact that the past sexual experience had been Johnny's didn't hold him back. Before long they were having intercourse.

"I did that because I love you, Dana," she said when they were finished. Her naked body was tight against his, her head on his chest. "Maybe you don't feel that strongly towards me now, but one day you will and I'll never deny you again." Then she rose, dressed, and slipped out the door.

Dana was more bewildered than pleased by the incident. He knew Jane had done it because of her intense feelings for him, yet he was unable to share her emotions. He cursed himself for being so uninvolved, yet he knew there was absolutely nothing he could do about it. He felt doomed forever to being a casual, insensitive observer of life, and he wanted so much to be a full participant in all its human pleasures and pains.

He was awakened for breakfast by the maid. Everything had returned to normal; Jane's hair was back in the bun and her glasses were set squarely upon her face. The only hint of the night before came when, after glancing about the room to make certain her parents and the kitchen staff were not looking, she kissed him gently.

Later that morning Dana was informed that the governor wanted to have a private talk with him. He was to go to the study at three o'clock.

Dana panicked when he heard the news. He was awed by the governor and frightened that the man might know what had gone on between himself and Jane. He wondered if he would be lectured about his conduct. His face went pale, he began to sweat, and he regretted having eaten lunch.

When the time came for the talk, Dana went to the study. The room was easily as imposing as the governor. It was richly paneled with a large desk and shelves loaded with books. He sat on an overstuffed leather chair and waited nervously.

The governor arrived a few minutes after three, sat down, and offered him a cigarette and a drink. Nervously, Dana accepted both.

The talk started in a casual way, the governor asking him about his background and his plans for the future. Then suddenly he asked the eternal question:

'What are your intentions towards my daughter?"

Dana felt his voice rising an octave; he hoped the change in pitch and the drink he had just spilled didn't make him appear too ridiculous. "My intentions?" he said. "I . . . uh . . . have a great fondness for Jane, Sir. I've liked her ever since I met her when she was dating Noel. You see, Noel and I were good friends and I thought he and Jane made a perfect couple."

The governor remained silent a moment, then he said, "My daughter tells me that she thinks she's in love with you." His voice was steady, his eyes calmly appraising Dana.

Well, if Jane said she loved him, Dana hurriedly replied, she was speaking from the top of her emotions and not from her heart. She was using him as a replacement for Noel, he was sure, and she didn't really know him well enough to be certain of her own mind. The transference of affection was a means of survival, in his opinion. It did not necessarily reflect her true feelings.

The governor seemed pleased by the response. He said he liked Dana and liked what he had heard, though he did not know him very well. He said he would offer no interference in their romance unless it became apparent, in time, that Dana was taking advantage of her feelings. He emphasized the fact that he did not wish to see his daughter marry at this time.

Dana explained that he also had no interest in seeing her married at that time. He did not share the feelings Jane had for him at the moment, and only time would tell what might develop.

The governor relaxed. He smiled, excused himself, and left the room. Dana, greatly relieved, joined Jane at the Olympic-sized, heated swimming pool in the backyard.

The following morning he packed to return to base, aware that he would have to end his relationship with her. She was far too serious about him for comfort; his own interest in her was relatively casual. Continuing to date her under the circumstances, he felt, would hardly be fair to her.

Several days passed before Dana decided to write her a letter. In it, he discussed his talk with the governor and his feeling that perhaps Jane was really transferring her affection for Noel to him, rather than getting to know him for his own sake. He told her she came from a world completely different from his and was not likely to be happy with him. He also said that his bizarre behavior changes had to be resolved before he could become serious about anyone. For all these reasons, he told her, it would be best if they stopped seeing or writing to one another.

She replied a short time later. Her letter professed deep love and included a solid gold St. Christopher's medal to keep him safe wherever he went. He never saw her again.

CHAPTER 11

While Dana and Johnny, through this period of my life, shared most of these romantic episodes, there was a time when Phil, too, was involved. To this day even the idea seems odd to me. Phil, after all, had appeared before only when, for some reason, it had seemed essential to keep the pressures of Dana's multiple existence from tearing him apart. He was always the rescuer when Johnny drove too recklessly or took off for an orgy of drinking and sex, as he would do frequently later in Dana's life. And even then, he seldom appeared for more than an hour or two, just long enough to accomplish his specific mission. The thought that he could actually nurture emotions of his own—indeed, the fact that he carried on a truly sensitive relationship that spanned a period of some weeks—seems foreign to his very nature.

Nevertheless it happened. One day, without warning, Phil fell deeply in love.

It was during a period when Dana was experiencing some difficulty with a knee that he had injured slightly in boot camp, then reinjured in the Korean War. He had to undergo surgery and spent several months recovering.

One of the first nights he was strong enough to leave the base, he got a pass and went to Baltimore to a nightclub. The show was a large revue with a chorus line, and at one point during it the girls went into the audience and danced with some of the men. Dana, sitting alone and in uniform, was a target for an attractive blonde dancer who took his hand and asked him to come forward. He only smiled, pointed to his cane, and explained that he was injured. The girl apologized and moved on to someone else.

When the show was over Dana was surprised to see the girl approach his table. "I just wanted to apologize for what I did during the show," she said, sitting down with him. "I hope I didn't cause you any embarrassment."

Dana talked with her a few minutes, assuring her she had done nothing wrong. Then the girl said, "You'd better buy me a drink. The management gets upset otherwise."

Dana ordered a rum and Coke for himself and was surprised when the girl told the waitress she wanted a champagne cocktail. He suddenly realized he was in a "clip joint," where the girls run up expensive bar tabs while sitting with the customers. He resented being used and told her so.

To his further surprise, the girl said she regretted using him that way. She explained that she was an actress who was down on her luck. She had tried to break into the theater in New York and had experienced just about every perverse aspect the business had to offer, including the indignities of the "casting couch." She was only twenty years old, but was having a hard time not becoming embittered. She had had hopes that she might do better in a smaller city like Baltimore, but so far had managed to land only the chorus job.

After a time Dana warmed toward the girl, and when she asked him if he wanted to go out with her for some Chinese food, he knew he wanted to. But he said he had very little money left, especially after paying for the champagne cocktail. "It's on me," she told him, taking his hand and urging him toward the door.

Dana enjoyed the dinner and, afterwards, drinks at an after-hours night spot frequented by Baltimore show people. After seeing the girl, Sally, to the residence hotel where she lived, Dana decided to remain in town for the night. She would not hear of his paying for a room in a hotel, however. The two of them spent the night together in her place.

While Dana liked the dancer and had thoroughly enjoyed their date, she was not the type of girl he would ever date a second time. Their relationship was over as far as he was concerned when he returned to camp the next day, even though he had written down her telephone number at breakfast. What he didn't realize was that Phil was also aware of Sally; in fact, he considered her the most desirable woman he had ever encountered.

The next time Dana was eligible for a pass he made plans to attend a show near the base with some of his fellow Marines. As he went to join them for the trip to town, he felt a tremendous depression and Phil took over. Phil immediately caught a bus to Baltimore and went to see Sally.

Sally and Phil soon became quite serious about each other. Although Dana did not know of Phil's existence, Phil was aware of Dana's; he knew, in fact, that the body he used was controlled by several different people, and he tried to explain this to Sally. He warned her that there might come a day when she would see him as a totally different person. He said that he could not marry her for that reason even though he did love her.

The romance between them went on for several weeks. Every time Dana got a pass, Phil took control of the body.

Then, one weekend, Phil was in the bar where Sally worked when he felt himself slipping into a depression of his own. A moment later he was gone and Dana was sitting in his place, bewildered at finding himself in the same club where he had first met Sally several weeks before. He glanced up and saw that the floor show was going on and that Sally was among the dancers. She looked at him, her face lighting up when their eyes made contact. He knew she recognized him, yet he had not been in the club since the night of their first meeting. He thought he must have made a very big impression on her then, yet he couldn't understand why he had bothered coming back. Whatever the reason, it completely escaped him—together with everything else that had occurred during the past several hours.

Sally came over to Dana's table the moment she was free. As she talked, he realized that she was in love with him. It also became obvious that he had spent other leaves with her, a confusing fact, which, however, at least let him know what had happened during some of his blackouts. Yet he felt no emotion toward the girl.

Eventually Dana and Sally went to her hotel room together. When they were alone she became somewhat distant, studying him as though studying a stranger. She knew Phil intimately and realized there was no connection between Phil and Dana.

"Is this the personality change you warned me about?" she asked. "Have you become that other person you said you might be some time?"

Whatever had happened during those lost weekends, Dana realized he must have told her about his problem. He must have explained that there were times he acted radically different, as if he were two separate people. He admitted to her that what she was asking was undoubtedly true. His personality must have changed if she remembered him differently from the way he was acting now.

Sally became quite upset. She told Dana he couldn't spend the night with her as he usually did. He would have to find someplace else to go. She didn't want him in her room anymore.

Dana left quietly. He felt badly about hurting Sally, though he had no memory of what their relationship must have been. He found a cheap room in another hotel and went to sleep. He would try to see her again in the morning. Perhaps he could learn more then.

But in the morning when Dana knocked at her door there was no response. He checked his watch and found it was close to the time she had to report for rehearsal at the club. He went there to find her but nobody there had seen her that morning either.

Puzzled, Dana returned to the hotel. He went to her door and knocked again. There was still no response. He tried the door handle and, to his surprise, it turned and opened.

The first thing that struck him once he was inside was how clean the suite looked. The living room was absolutely spotless. Although Sally was by nature a fairly neat person, this went beyond simple neatness. Dana realized it would have taken her several hours to straighten everything so perfectly.

He walked to the bedroom door and pushed it open. Sally was lying in the bed, an empty bottle of barbiturates beside her. There was a note propped on the table next to the bed. It read:

"To A Man Who Is Not:

"I have loved once and have been loved once. I can not love again. I don't know where you have gone. This is the only way I know of to find you."

It was signed "Sally."

Dana checked to see if she was still alive. Her body was cold, and there was a slight stiffness in her limbs. She had been dead for some time.

But even this discovery didn't upset Dana. It was unpleasant, but he was incapable of feeling a sense of loss. He accepted it as he accepted everything else.

He left the room, closed the door, and went back to the club. There he told the manager that he had been unable to reach Sally on the hotel telephone, and that perhaps someone should go across the street and use the hotel's pass key to get into her room. Then he went to the bus station and returned to base.

Whatever grief Phil may have experienced is not known. All that is certain is that he kept it to himself, suffering quietly in the recess of my mind that he called home.

CHAPTER 12

On January 28, 1954, Dana received his honorable discharge from the U.S. Marines and caught a plane that would take him back to his father's home in California.

The last five months of his enlistment had passed quickly, with a minimum of trouble from both Johnny and Peter. Only once, in fact, had Johnny emerged for more than an hour or two. That incident had occurred during a thirty-day leave Dana had taken some months earlier during his recovery from knee surgery. Johnny had suddenly taken over, located the revolver Dana had brought back from Korea, and spent an afternoon terrorizing his old friend Jack Lesley and Jack's girl Ruby with it. He had finally ended up having intercourse with Ruby—something neither she nor Jack seemed to object to very much—then laughing the whole matter off as a joke. Throughout the rest of his leave Ruby continued to call Dana, much to his confusion, and to invite him to come back for another visit.

It was during these last months of Dana's Marine career, too, that Johnny first developed a habit that was to plague Dana for the next twenty years. For some reason Johnny hated the idea that Dana exercised primary control over the body. He also resented the fact that Dana was completely unaware of him. As a result he decided to provide Dana with a constant reminder of his existence. Every time he was in charge and felt himself losing control, he would take the last few minutes to place a lighted cigarette against his arm, submerging before the pain began to mount. Dana would suddenly regain consciousness and find himself with a throbbing, blistering sore on his arm and no idea at all of how it got there.

Over the years Johnny would burn Dana in much the same way an old-time Western gunfighter might notch his gun butt each time he killed an opponent in a shoot-out. The burns were visible signs of his presence and his power. As Johnny himself was to explain later, "They're just my way of saying, 'Fuck you!'" But for many years Dana remained puzzled over their meaning.

And now, at long last, he was finished with the Marines, going back to California for good. The return home proved more pleasant than he had expected. His father and Brenda had had a baby girl who was already six months old. Brenda was spending more time at home, and even Dana's father seemed to be trying to be more of a parent than he had been the first time around. Dana felt a sense of family for the first time in years. It was a pleasant feeling.

The first night home, his father told Dana of his plans for the future. Dana was to come into the store at the bottom, working in the warehouse, stocking merchandise and preparing appliances for delivery. As he learned the business he would be advanced quickly. Eventually he would become a full partner with an income equal to his father's $60,000 to $70,000 a year. However, his income at first would be just $75 a week.

Dana was happy about the job and enthusiastic about the money he would be making, despite the fact that he was expected to pay Brenda $25 a week for his room and board. He felt that for the first time in his life he was going to be able to please his father. And he looked forward to the chance to prove his abilities in the appliance business.

To make commuting a little easier, his father gave Dana a 1950 Ford Coupe as a coming-home present. With the job, the car, and the few hundred dollars he had saved in the Marines, Dana felt on top of the world.

"That chickenshit's been home twenty-four hours and he hasn't celebrated getting out of that damned Marine Corps yet," thought Johnny as he took control the second evening Dana was home. Since he was in the car, he immediately pulled off the road at a bar. He took four drinks in a row, astounding the bartender as he gulped one after the other, then walked out without showing any effects of the alcohol.

He drove toward Oakland, thinking he would stop to see Ellen in her new apartment there. He knew she'd be glad to see him no matter how unexpected the visit; he hadn't had a good lay since Ruby. Hell, he was going to have a good time!

Noticing a bar on the outskirts of Oakland, Johnny decided not to pass it without having a little more libation. He consumed two more drinks in moments.

He returned to the car and looked out at the light of the Oakland hills. "Let's see what kind of car Dana's son-of-a-bitch father gave him," he thought, as he drove into the city. He accelerated quickly, taking the hills as fast as the car would go.

Between the roller-coaster effect of the streets and the low-powered engine, Johnny quickly found himself bored. He let his eyes wander a moment and accidentally struck a bump. It was not a severe jolt but it caught him unprepared while the car was moving at eighty miles an hour through a residential area; he immediately lost control.

The car began sliding sideways, sideswiping ten parked cars in a row. He turned the wheel sharply and the vehicle cut across a front lawn, digging deep ruts into the ground.

He brought the car back on the street, then careened across another yard and slammed into a front porch. The car flipped onto its side, slid a few feet, and stopped, the wheels spinning in the air. Johnny was thrown out the door.

"Hell, that's celebrating!" said Johnny, glancing around before submerging so that Dana would be the one to face the police he was certain the neighbors had called.

Dana found himself sitting in the middle of someone's yard. His eyes took a moment to accustom themselves to the dark. He didn't know where he was or how he had gotten there.

A crowd began to form in the yard as people rushed to see what had caused all the noise. Then, for the first time, Dana noticed the car on its side. He could feel the effects of the alcohol Johnny had been drinking, but he had no memory of stopping at a bar. He wondered where he was and just how the accident had happened.

Dana got shakily to his feet as a patrol car and ambulance pulled to the curb. His clothing was torn and his back was sore from the slide across the grass, but he wasn't seriously hurt and he told the police the ambulance was unnecessary.

He was arrested and convicted of drunk driving for Johnny's action. His license was suspended for thirty days and he was fined $180. It proved to be the first of many such arrests.

His father was surprisingly understanding about it. He blamed the incident on an emotional letdown after being released from the service. He said he could understand Dana's celebrating and having too much to drink. He also said he could feel free to drive in their immediate community because he was a police commissioner now and none of the officers would arrest his son.

A few days later Dana learned that one of his friends was moving out of state. He and several other of the young man's friends decided to throw a party for him in Dana's father's house. It was at that party that Dana first met a girl named Ann O'Reilly, who had been dating Ralph Potter more or less regularly for the past few months. She lacked the extreme good looks and almost animal sex appeal that Ellen possessed, but something about her attracted Dana to her more than to any other girl he had ever met. Throughout the evening he spent as much time as possible talking with her, though she didn't register much interest. Part of the problem proved to be that she thought Dana and Ellen were engaged. As a joke, Ellen had been introduced as Dana's fiancee, but no one had bothered to tell Ann it wasn't true.

Ellen had what she considered a rather boring time that night. Dana was his usual quiet self during the party, his only animation seeming to come when he talked with Ann. To make matters worse for Ellen, when she spent the night at Dana'a house she found his lovemaking totally unsatisfactory. She had been looking forward to the violent passion of Johnny; his brutal approach was what aroused her. Dana seemed almost mechanical, and she regretted that he was in such a somber mood.

Dana met Ann again the following afternoon. She, Ralph, and Jack Lesley came over to help clean up after the party, then the four of them went cruising on a nearby waterway on the boat Dana's father and Brenda owned.

Ann remained very much in Dana's thoughts. He finally got the nerve to call her after he started working in his father's store. Ann wanted nothing to do with him, however. Thinking he was engaged to someone else, she had no desire to come between them. She refused to answer the telephone or let him come over and talk with her.

But Dana was not about to be put off. After a half dozen unanswered calls, he looked up her address and wrote her a letter. He explained that the talk of an engagement had been a joke, that he was not seriously involved with anyone. He told her he was sorry she was so serious about Ralph because, had they met earlier, things might have worked out quite differently for them. He said that perhaps some of their differences could be resolved if she would only talk with him on the telephone.

Ann was intrigued by the letter, even though she

thought Dana was handing her a line. However, it did put him in a slightly different light, and when he called her again she decided to talk with him.

Dana convinced her this time to give him a date of sorts. Since she had to babysit for one of her married friends, she agreed to let Dana accompany her on the job. It would only be until ten o'clock, and her friend was going to drive her home, but if Dana felt he had to see her, well then this would have to do.

The brief date went fairly well. Ann wasn't particularly impressed with him, though she liked him more than she thought she would. She had thought he might be arrogant and overly confident, coming from a wealthy family and having spent the last few years in the Marines, but her concerns proved groundless. She even let him drive her home that night, but when he tried to kiss her she turned her cheek, an action that made Dana think he hadn't made the impression he had hoped for.

He was nervous when he called her about the possibility of going to a drive-in movie the following weekend.

To his surprise, however, she said she would go—provided she could pick the movie. Naturally he agreed.

That Friday night when Dana picked her up, he was immediately informed that her parents were strict about the hours she kept, since she was only recently out of high school and still living at home. She had to be in by 10 on weekdays and midnight on weekends, without exception. Dana said he would abide by her parents' wishes.

The second date went better than the first. They enjoyed each other's company and she told him she would like to go out with him again. During the next few months they began seeing each other often.

Ellen, meanwhile, was still very much in Dana's life, a fact that was soon to have serious repercussions. She had come from a background that had left her insecure about herself and her future. As she got to know Dana's father and Brenda, she became intrigued by their wealth. Their house overlooked the ocean and they owned a boat as well as two Cadillacs. She felt that if she married their son, she would have financial security for the rest of her life.

Yet she was obviously disappointed with Dana. When they made love it was almost as though he was following a step-by-step chart. Johnny had torn off her clothes and thrown her around, letting her know that if she failed to submit he would go ahead and rape her. It was Johnny who excited her. Nevertheless she came to the decision that she would rather settle for less-than-satisfactory sex with Dana than lose the security of his family's appliance business. She soon began a concentrated attack to get Dana to propose.

Dana simply wasn't interested in Ellen, especially since he had met Ann. However, his father and Brenda were quite taken with her. They thought she was ideal for their son and frequently invited her to dinner. They also made unkind remarks about Ann, trying to tear her down in Dana's eyes.

At one point his father went so far as to make Ellen a part of the business. He arranged a promotional stunt in which he sent her out to various restaurants and shopping centers in the city. Called "The Frigidaire Queen," she carried a gift certificate in her purse that was good for a new Frigidaire refrigerator. The idea behind the promotion was for someone to find her and ask her if she was the Frigidaire Queen. Whoever did would get the certificate and the appliance. It was an extremely successful promotion. Soon everyone in town was walking up to pretty girls everywhere and asking them if they were the queen. When Ellen was finally discovered, the local paper even ran her picture on the front page.

During this period Johnny showed the only hint of emotion he ever displayed. He became jealous of Ellen and angry that she was willing to marry Dana, even though Dana didn't turn her on the way Johnny did. He decided finally to have it out with her.

Dana was reading quietly at home that night. Suddenly a wave of depression hit him and Johnny slammed the book down, walked to the kitchen, took several shots of liquor, and walked out of the house. He drove to Ellen's apartment and pounded on her door until she answered it.

"Dana, what brings you over here?"

Johnny roughly pushed her aside, striding into the living room. She was immediately turned on by the action; she closed and double-locked the door. "I see you've got that special spark of yours back," she said, stroking his arm.

"You're damned right, baby," he said, his lip curled in a half smile. His body was tense and his eyes wild. He kissed her roughly, then told her to get him a drink.

"Anything you want," she said. She brought each of them a glass of liquor, sipping hers slowly while he gulped his down. He poured himself a second glassful, swallowed it, then grabbed her by the arms.

"I'm going to show you what it's like to be balled by an expert," he told her, angrily tearing off her clothes. Ellen offered no resistance, her face showing the pleasure she found in his abuse. They made love on the couch, their clothes strewn about the room.

"Wow!" she said. "Now that's the man I've been looking for all these weeks."

Johnny grabbed her wrist, bending her arm back until it hurt. "That's why I'm here, you stupid bitch! I don't want you coming around the house and calling Dana all the time. I'm sick of the way you hang around there. If I catch you pestering him again, I'll beat the shit out of you. Do you understand?"

Ellen didn't understand at all, but she said she'd do whatever he wanted. She liked the violence when it involved sex, but he was hurting her for some other reason now and that scared her.

"You damn well better. If you don't I'm going to beat the hell out of you so bad that nobody's ever going to want you again!" He released her arm, pushing her back against the couch. Then he got dressed and drove back to Dana's house. He took another drink in the kitchen, then walked upstairs to the room where Dana had been sitting, returned to the chair, and let Dana take control. He was satisfied that *his* girl wouldn't throw herself at Dana again.

Dana felt strange, sitting in the same chair he had been in before without having advanced very far in his book. He thought he might have dozed off, yet he was aware that there was alcohol in his body and he was sure he hadn't had a drink. Normally when he had amnesia he found himself in a strange location; this time there wasn't a single clue as to what had occurred.

Ann and Dana continued to date with ever-increasing frequency, and after a few months they decided to go steady. Marriage was still not a serious consideration, although they knew they'd rather be together than with anyone else.

Then Dana's father threw one of the parties that were beginning to make him famous in his community. The parties began on Friday night and didn't end until sometime Sunday afternoon.

The guest list for one of his typical parties included the Mayor and the Chief of Police, as well as a Mafia don whose money came from several legitimate restaurants and the prostitutes in one of the larger California cities. The shoe shine man who worked in a barber shop down the street from the appliance store sometimes came, as did his friends. There were social leaders and semi-winos whom Dana's father had met while bar-hopping. The butcher usually came and brought enough meat with him to feed the entire crowd. Many of the guests arrived on luxury boats they tied up at the dock behind the house, others drove Cadillacs, and still others came in beat-up junk heaps that barely ran. Those who couldn't afford cars walked or took the bus.

The first night of this particular party was all Johnny's. He wasn't belligerent, he was just happy to be able to eat and drink anything he wanted. The only time he became aggressive was when he met a German stewardess who was married to an airline pilot. He managed to get her away from her husband and took her on a boat, where they had sex together. By early Saturday morning, however, he had had his fill of the party. He went to bed and Dana awakened in his place. He immediately called Ann and invited her to be his date that night. Ralph Potter and his date were also attending, so the four would be able to have fun together.

Dana's father met Ann for the first time that night, though he had known for months that Dana was dating her. He looked her over, then said rather coldly, "You don't know what you're getting yourself into. My son's changeable and can be a wild bastard!" Not understanding what he meant, she quickly forgot the remark.

After introducing Ann to the other guests, Dana suggested that Ralph and his date join them on the boat. They brought along a six-pack of beer and soft drinks, started the boat, and pulled away from the dock.

When the boat reached the middle of the waterway behind the house, they decided to drop anchor and just sit around, talking. After a half hour or so Dana had to go below to use the bathroom. He was just washing his hands when Johnny decided it was time for him to take charge. He knew there was liquor in a locker down below; he found the bottle, quickly took four shots of booze, and called to Ann, asking her to come below. The moment she was out of sight of Ralph and his date, Johnny caught hold of her and began to remove her clothes.

Ann was shocked by his behavior and pushed him away. "Are you crazy or something?" she asked.

Laughing, Johnny followed her topside and asked Ralph to give him a beer. He drank it down and tossed the can into the water.

The beer only increased his amorous desire. He walked over to Ann and gave her a hard kiss, at the same time letting his hands roam freely over her body. She pushed him back, a response that set him laughing again.

Ann was angry. No matter how much she cared for Dana, she wasn't going to be mistreated and then mocked by him. She suddenly pushed him again as hard as she could, sending him over the boat's railing.

"Stupid bitch!" thought Johnny, wet and sputtering. "The chickenshit can have her!" He turned control back to Dana, who found himself floundering in the water, looking up in confusion at the boat.

"I hope you drown!" said Ann, angrily, looking over the side. "You no-good. . . . "

"Hey, I don't know what I did but I'm sorry," shouted Dana. He was treading water, dumbfounded by all that had happened. "Somebody pull me out of here."

Ralph leaned over the side and helped him climb back into the boat. Ann glared at him, her eyes blazing. "You just better not do anything like that ever again or we're through!" she said angrily.

Dana apologized and said he didn't know what had gotten into him.

"You acted as if you had gotten into some booze when you were down below," she said.

"I did have a couple of shots," Dana admitted. He knew that liquor was kept there, but he also knew that he hadn't taken any of it. Still, if claiming that he had been drinking would soothe Ann, he was willing to lie a little. "I guess it made me get a little out of hand. I'm sorry for the way I acted."

She accepted this apology, but the afternoon had been ruined for all of them. They pulled anchor and headed back to the dock.

The incident on the boat hurt Dana's relations with Ann only for a few days. By the end of the following week they were going together again. Ann, in fact, had gotten into the habit of dropping by the warehouse with a bagged lunch for him. Brenda refused to fix him a lunch and he couldn't afford to eat out. Ann also said she would start doing his laundry for him because, though his father hired a maid, nobody ever bothered taking care of Dana's clothing.

During this period Peter was carefully studying Ann. He knew that whomever Dana married would be an integral part of his own life, so he was naturally curious. He came to the conclusion that he liked Ann and would be proud to have her as Dana's wife. He also was aware that because of Dana's limited emotional range, he would be unable fully to declare his love for her.

Peter began taking control at night, determined to influence Dana's decision. He wrote poems of love—poems he left behind for Dana to discover. They were signed only with the initial "P," and Dana never understood how they came about. However, he read them and they helped him arrive at a decision. He would propose marriage to Ann.

His father always gave a Fourth of July picnic for his employees, held in a secluded park in the hills above the city. The area was cool and pleasant, with plenty of room for the usual games.

On July 4, 1954, Dana was to pick up Ann and take her to the picnic at noon. He had also agreed to make an earlier trip to the grounds at 8:30 that morning to help his father and Brenda get everything prepared.

Dana was just getting ready to leave in his car that morning when he remembered that his camera was still inside the house. He wanted to take it to the picnic and didn't think he'd be returning home before going to pick up Ann. He went back into the house to get it.

He always kept the camera in a desk drawer in his room. Before he could open the drawer he blacked out and Peter took control.

Peter was excited. He knew Dana was going to see Ann and that he was very likely to propose to her. He also knew that Dana had never expressed his love for her, something Peter felt he should correct. He feared that unless Ann knew that Dana really loved her, she might refuse the proposal.

Peter took a piece of paper and began composing a poem. He told Ann that she was like a gift of love for Dana. He said he was pleased with Dana's good fortune, though saddened by the pain he knew Dana would cause her. He called her an "angel of love."

When he had finished, he went rushing from the house, thinking excitedly as he backed out of the drive about her probable reaction. He didn't bother concentrating on where he was going and managed to scrape one of the car's fenders against a fencepost.

He arrived at Ann's house at 10:30. He would have arrived even sooner but he had gotten lost along the way. He had never before paid much attention to the route during the months Dana and Ann were courting.

He came to a jerky stop, scraping the car's tires against the curb, then bounded out of the car and loped up to the house. His body seemed to move with all the grace of a bouncing ping-pong ball.

"What are you doing here?" asked Ann, answering his knock. She noticed that his eyes were wider and shinier than usual. His boyish grin, too, looked rather silly on his normally serious face. She suspected he was drunk. "You're early."

"I got something I want to show you," said Peter. His voice was that of an enthusiastic child and it startled Ann. He seemed to be shaking from excitement, as though he would explode at any moment. Peter was used to putting his emotions into writing rather than expressing them verbally, yet he had to tell Ann what he thought of her and why she was so special to Dana. He had to face her and let her see his poem, and it was all so embarrassing.

"You've been drinking again," said Ann coldly.

"No! No! No!" he said, his enthusiasm only slightly dampened by her response. "I haven't been drinking. I just got something to show you. I got something in the car. It's important. I gotta show you. I gotta show you!" His face was flushed from the excitement and he giggled nervously. He was like a small boy who is so embarrassed he hides, trembling, behind his mother's skirt.

Ann was convinced that Dana was drunk, and she was determined to check his breath at the first opportunity.

Peter took her hand and hurried her toward the car. He seemed almost to be skipping, forcing her to move quickly to keep up with him. Whatever he had to show her, it must be important, she thought.

Peter opened the door on the passenger side and told Ann to get inside. "No," she said, firmly. "I'm not ready to go anywhere with you. You said you wouldn't come by here till noon. That's an hour and a half from now."

"No, you don't understand. We're not going anywhere. I'm just going to show you something. Get in! Get in!" Peter was suddenly scared. He realized that the only reason she was going along with him was that she thought he was Dana. If she recognized that he was actually a different person she might go back inside the house. He had to show her the poem because it would reveal to her the feelings that Dana himself could never express. It would let her know how everyone but that bad Johnny really felt about her. She just had to get inside!

With Ann finally on the seat beside him, Peter reached into his coat pocket and took out the poem. He read it aloud, letting her hold it when he was through.

"Is that what was so important that you had to come right over to my house? That's the craziest poem I've ever heard," Ann said. "Who are all those people talking in the poem? And why do you keep referring to yourself as though it's not really you talking?"

Peter said nothing. He swallowed painfully.

"And that line about being an angel. Are you saying you think I'm some kind of angel and that you love me? That's very sweet—but was it necessary to act so strangely in order to tell me?"

Peter was aghast. He realized he had made a fool of himself. Instead of improving Dana's relationship with Ann by expressing feelings of love, he had somehow made Ann upset with him. He didn't know what to say. He finally blurted, "You're an angel and I'll pick you up at noon."

Ann leaned over to kiss him, hoping as she did so to detect any trace of alcohol. But Peter quickly moved out of the way, blushing. He had never kissed a girl in his whole life, and he didn't think he ever would. Kissing was all right for Dana but not for Peter Pan. He liked Ann, yet he would not get involved in any of that.

Ann got out of the car, walked around to the driver's side, and caught Peter off his guard. She managed to give him a light kiss through the open window, and he blushed again. She also satisfied herself that he had not been drinking.

She had mixed emotions when she went back inside the house. She was bothered by the fact that Dana had seemed about as mature as a seven-year-old. Then she thought about what he had written and the fact that it was the first time she had ever heard him express words of love for her. The thought excited her, for she did love Dana, and the poem told her that he loved her as well.

Dana arrived at Ann's house exactly at noon, as originally planned. He came to a smooth stop in front of the curb and walked to her door. His eyes were dull compared with Peter's and he lacked Peter's exuberant manner.

Ann immediately noticed the change in him but assumed he was simply back to normal. He didn't mention having seen her earlier in the day or having read her a poem. She thought he was ashamed of the way he had acted, not knowing that he was totally unaware of Peter's actions. She decided not to bring up the subject unless he did.

The picnic was in full swing when Dana and Ann arrived. Children were running about, laughing. People were eating hot dogs, drinking lemonade, and playing games. Everywhere there were high spirits. Only Dana remained his usual dull self, unable to throw himself into the activities. As he watched the others, it was obvious that he preferred to be somewhere else.

"You're not letting yourself have fun," said Ann.

Dana didn't respond. He watched the people at play and wondered what it was that enabled them to let go like that. One girl was giggling and running from her laughing boy friend. He thought it would be nice to feel like that, even though he didn't know just what the feeling might be. He just recognized that others seemed to be able to experience life to a greater degree than he could. That was the way he had been all his life. He'd just have to live with it. He hoped Ann would understand.

"Do you want to leave?" Ann asked him.

"No. I promised my father I'd stay till the end so I could help with the clean-up."

"I just wish you were having a better time."

Dana said nothing. He did, too. For Ann's sake, even if not for his own. He had begun to wonder whether he was even being fair with her, thinking that she might want to spend a lifetime with someone as dull as he.

But the following day Phil and Peter began working on Dana anyway, trying to get him to propose. They felt that Ann was the perfect girl for him. Dana was aware of the voices, though again he could not make out the specific words. He sensed the message the others were attempting to tell him, even though he tried to ignore the sounds inside his head. During his noon lunch break he went to a local jeweler and purchased an engagement ring and a wedding ring with a solitaire diamond.

Dana returned to work, nervously glancing at the clock to see when he could leave. As soon as quitting time came around he called Ann, telling her there was something he had to tell her. Apparently the excitement in his voice reminded her a little of Peter and she commented, "You mean you're going to read me another poem? Can't that wait until our next date?"

Dana was confused. "What do you mean 'read you another poem?' I don't know what you're talking about."

"Forget it," she said. "It's nothing."

"I'm serious about wanting to talk with you. Can we go out tonight? I'll have you home by 10."

Ann agreed. He picked her up and together they drove to the nearby airport, parking on a field overlooking the landing strip. Dana tossed the box of rings into her lap and rather awkwardly said, "Let's get married."

Ann was thrilled, despite Dana's casual attitude. She would have liked him to be more romantic, but then she knew he simply wasn't that kind of man. She smiled and said, "This isn't exactly the way I expected to be proposed to —just throwing me a box of rings."

Dana looked down and said, "I'm sorry I'm so clumsy.

This is an awkward thing for me, too."

Ann opened the box and looked at the rings. "Why don't you take the engagement ring and slip it on my finger?" she said.

Dana said excitedly, "Does that mean you'll marry me?"

"Yes," she said softly as Dana pushed the ring on her hand. Then she put her arms around his neck, pulled him close, and kissed him.

It was nearing 10 as Dana took her home. He felt both relief and happiness. The woman he loved as much as he could love anyone was actually willing to be his wife.

CHAPTER 13

Several days after the engagement, Dana had a dinner date with Ann. He got dressed, walked down the stairs, and blacked out. For some reason, Johnny had decided to pick Ann up in Dana's place. He drove over to the house and began hitting the horn.

Ann was surprised by the sound of the car horn. Dana always came to the door to get her. His formal politeness was one of the things she loved about him.

"Aren't you coming to the house?" Ann called out to him.

"No. Come on. I'm waiting in the car." The bitch wasn't worth the bother.

Ann realized that something was wrong with Dana the moment she stepped into the car. His appearance, tone of voice, and attitude were so unlike the Dana she loved.

Johnny told Ann that he had broken the news of their engagement to his father. Actually he had not—nor had Dana. His father and Brenda still had hopes that Dana would marry Ellen—this even despite the fact that Ellen had recently married another man. The man, Dana's old

friend Larry Cardwell, was working as a lowly X-ray technician, however, and they felt that he could never provide
Ellen with the luxuries she seemed to desire. As a result
they were still making every effort to split Dana and Ann;
they felt they would never be happy with Ann as a daugh-
ter-in-law.

And now, with a perfectly straight face, Johnny told
Ann that his father approved of their engagement and
wanted to talk with them together about their plans. Ann
was nervous about the prospect and assumed that Dana's
odd attitude only reflected his own fear.

Apparently Johnny thought putting his father and Ann
in the same room together, when his father had not been
told about the engagement, would be very funny. When
they reached the house, Johnny left Ann in the living
room, then told his father that she wanted to talk with
him. His father came out and sat down with her, at which
point Johnny announced he was going out to buy some cigarettes. "You two talk until I get back," he said and
headed for the nearest bar. He had two drinks, then submerged and let Dana take control.

Meanwhile, in the house, Ann was chattering away
about the beautiful engagement ring, about how happy she
was and about all the other things a bride-to-be has on her
mind. Her nervousness made the words flow, but she believed that all she was doing was telling Dana's father
things that he had already been told.

Dana's father sat listening, his face growing increasingly somber. "Tell me the truth, Ann. Are you pregnant?"
His voice was cold.

"What do you mean?" she asked, shocked.

"Did my son get you pregnant? Is that why he got you
those rings? What did he do, take you to a motel one night?
He's a wild bastard. It wouldn't surprise me in the least."

Ann protested that she wasn't pregnant and had never
done anything to get pregnant. Still Dana's father continued to question her. He finally came to the conclusion
that she was telling the truth, though that knowledge

didn't seem to offer him much comfort. A pregnancy could be terminated by abortion. But a marriage because two people really cared about each other . . . that was far worse.

He decided finally to call Brenda into the room and share the news with her. Perhaps a woman could find words more appropriate to the situation.

Brenda was hardly more thrilled than Dana's father. She listened to the news, looked at the ring, then said abruptly, "I guess that little thing was all Dana could afford." As if to emphasize her attitude, she nonchalantly twisted the $7,000 diamond ring on her own finger.

Back in the bar, Dana was quite upset when he realized what time it was. He had a date with Ann and somehow he had gone to get a drink instead of picking her up. He rushed out to his car and drove to her house, hoping she'd forgive him.

"You came for Ann?" asked her brother, surprised to see Dana there. "But you were just here to pick her up an hour ago. Isn't she with you?"

"Yes," said Dana, quickly covering up. "This is all part of a joke. Don't worry about it. Don't say anything. It's all okay." Smiling but perturbed, he returned to the car. He would go back to his house. Perhaps he had left her there.

"Boy, that was a long way to go for a pack of cigarettes," said Ann as he entered the living room. "What did you do, go to Turkey?" She was fuming.

Dana was relieved to see her. "I got hung up in conversation with someone," he replied. "I'm sorry." He had no idea how Ann had gotten there or why he had left her with his parents.

"That sure was a mean trick you played on me," Ann continued, angrily. "I thought you had discussed our engagement with your father. I was showing him the ring and rattling on about our wedding plans and he didn't have the slightest idea what I was talking about."

Dana was embarrassed by the position he had apparently put Ann in, yet he had run out of excuses. Finally he just blurted, "We're running a little late. Maybe we should go off to dinner." Ann sighed, and they went out to his car.

"Why did you do a thing like that?" she demanded, her eyes blazing. "Why did you dump me off at your father's house and tell me that he knew all about us?"

Dana felt like crawling through the floor. He hated to lie, especially to Ann, but he couldn't yet find the strength to tell her the truth about his blackouts and amnesia spells. They were too frightening even for him to face, and he didn't want to lose the most important person ever to enter his life. "I know my father," he said, cursing himself for his dishonesty. "That was the only way I could really tell him about us and be sure he would accept it."

Ann resented the approach he had taken but grew calmer about it as time passed. The rest of the evening went comparatively well, and Dana once again managed to put his anguish out of his mind.

But when he returned home later that evening his father questioned him just as he had Ann. "You were out foolin' around in some motel and you got caught, didn't you?" he demanded. "You don't have to marry her just because you got her pregnant, you know. We're living in a time when they can fix that sort of thing."

Dana, too, insisted that there was no pregnancy and no problem. They just wanted to be married. It was their choice, made without pressure of any kind.

"You mean you *want* to marry that little nothing?" asked Brenda, showing her dismay. "You let someone like Ellen slip through your fingers so you can propose to *her?*" She looked away, as if she were in the presence of someone who was simply beyond hope.

"Let's not worry about it," said Dana's father. "Ann said they want a September wedding. That's a few months off. He'll come to his senses by then."

Shortly afterward Dana received a promotion. He was taken out of the warehouse and put on the sales floor of the main store. It was a glamorous position where he might be able to meet other women. He was also to accompany his father on buying trips to San Francisco, where he met some of his father's most important and influential friends. Apparently his father felt that if Dana was exposed to the beautiful people of the world, he would find Ann comparatively dull.

Dana was an ineffective salesman at first. He was quiet and introverted, characteristics that did not make for success in the business. He had trouble smiling at people, too, especially strangers. His voice was a monotone and he lacked the dramatic flare necessary for selling.

But his father felt that he had to turn Dana into a top producer, so he began giving him lessons in salesmanship. He made Dana practice sales pitches standing in front of a mirror and working on his smile for an hour at a time. He taught him to vary the pitch of his voice, how to greet a customer, how to close a sale.

Dana's desire to please his father gradually overcame his shyness. He tried hard to learn and caught on fairly quickly. Within two months he was every bit the equal of the professional salesmen on the staff.

His father was a firm believer in rewarding success —but only as much as he absolutely had to. He raised Dana's weekly pay from the $85 he had been getting to $125. This increase was far less than it appeared to be, however. The other salesmen were paid on commission; those who sold as well as Dana were taking home more than $200 a week.

In August Johnny decided to break Dana's engagement with Ann, once and for all. He could see no sense in having her around all the time, so he thought he would do something to get her angry.

He chose a day on which Dana and Ann were taking a long drive to southern California to visit her brother and sister-in-law. They decided while there to go on into Mexico for the day, a trip Johnny felt was ideal for him. He took over as they went across the border.

Johnny decided he wanted some Tequila and all the other liquid pleasures unique to the area. Despite her protests, he began dragging Ann from one cheap bar to another.

"So the bitch doesn't want to have fun?" Johnny snarled angrily. "What the hell good are you if you never try to get a few kicks?"

Ann finally got Johnny back in the car and they left Mexico, traveling at 100 miles an hour through California. He refused to say a word to her. His eyes were cold and glaring as he concentrated on the road ahead, weaving in and out of the traffic.

When he was thirty miles from where Ann lived he decided he had had enough of her for that day. He let Dana take over.

Dana expressed no surprise at finding himself going north instead of south. He eased his foot off the gas until the car was traveling at a safe, legal speed, then he began talking as though nothing had happened. His actions confused Ann, who finally decided that he wanted to let her know he was sorry for the way he had acted, even though he couldn't express it in so many words. She later forgot about the incident, and Johnny didn't appear before her again until well after the wedding.

They were married in a big church ceremony. Ann's family was large, and 300 guests attended the reception. Dana's father invited all the government officials, Mafia leaders, and other influential people he knew. Even though it was quite a celebration, Johnny never bothered to come out. He apparently wanted no part of a wedding, even with liquor being served.

Dana's father gave him his credit cards for hotels in Las Vegas and Reno so that he and Ann could honeymoon there without expense. He also promised the couple $1,000 in cash—$500 to be paid before they left on their honeymoon and $500 after they returned. He gave them the first half but conveniently forgot the rest—they never saw the second $500.

Ann, who had led a fairly sheltered life, had a little trouble adjusting to her new marital status while on the honeymoon. The couple stayed at the fanciest hotel in Reno, enjoying the gambling and the sights until very late. They got to bed early in the morning, then decided they were hungry. "Why don't we call room service," suggested Dana. "I'd like a hot fudge sundae."

"Do you think we can get one at this time of night?" asked Ann.

"Reno's a city that lives twenty-four hours a day. You can get anything at any time," said Dana. He called room service. They didn't have hot fudge sundaes available from the hotel at that hour, the voice on the telephone said, but they were certain they could get them if the gentleman didn't mind waiting.

Forty-five minutes later there was a knock at the door. "Room service," said the voice outside.

Ann jumped out of bed. "This is embarrassing. Help me make the bed," she whispered excitedly.

"What for?"

"Just help me make the bed."

"Just a minute," said Dana to the door. He helped Ann make up the bed. Then she snatched up all her belongings and locked herself in the bathroom while Dana slipped on his pants and opened the door.

"I brought your hot fudge sundaes," said the man. He glanced about the room, noticing that the bed was apparently untouched. He could see Dana's bags but there was no sign of anyone else staying there. "You did order *two* hot fudge sundaes?" he asked, hesitantly.

"Yes," said Dana, accepting the sundaes. He tipped the man and closed the door.

Then he crossed the room and knocked on the bathroom door. "He's gone. You can come out now."

Ann said she had never been in a hotel room with a man before and that she was embarrassed, that's all. It all still felt a little strange to her. They both got back into bed to eat the ice cream.

Several hours later, hungry again, they decided to order breakfast in bed rather than going out to a restaurant.

They ordered bacon, eggs, hot cakes, juice—the works. Then they waited for the delivery.

It was a repeat of what had happened with the ice cream order. When the man knocked at the door, Ann insisted on making the bed and taking her belongings into the bathroom.

The same person who brought the sundaes brought the two large breakfast orders. Again his eyes searched the room and again he saw an apparently untouched bed and the belongings of just one person. "Do I have this order right?" he asked. "There are two breakfasts?"

Dana said he had brought the order exactly as it had been placed. The man accepted the tip, shook his head, and walked out the door. Even in Reno, this had been a new experience for him.

The couple's first home, a furnished three-room basement apartment, proved unpleasant when Ann and Dana returned from their honeymoon. It was typical of many basements in the area—constantly damp and mildewed. After several months they decided to take an apartment in a converted attic. It was fairly well furnished but lacked appliances.

Dana felt that buying appliances would be no problem since his father was the biggest dealer in town. He asked him about getting the appliances at a wholesale price. His father, however, insisted on making a profit on everything he sold, even when his only son was involved. He told Dana that he would have to pay the same price as the other salesmen—wholesale plus twenty percent. The twenty percent represented his father's profit.

Dana resented his father's lack of generosity but was willing to go along. It was still cheaper than buying anywhere else. Then suddenly his father apparently had a change of heart. "Tell you what I'll do," he said. "I'll give you enough appliances to get you by without purchasing anything right now."

Dana was overwhelmed by what seemed to be a generous offer. He tried to thank him, but his father merely shrugged his gratitude off. Dana was not to worry about what appliances he would be getting, he told him. Everything would be delivered to the house and he could inspect it there.

In fact, Dana's need merely provided his father with a handy excuse to clear out some of the junk that had accumulated over the years. He collected all the barely working, out-of-date merchandise he had and gave it to Dana.

The refrigerator was the first shock. It was a General Electric with the condenser at the top—a unit roughly thirty years old. Washing machines had been automatic for years but Dana's father managed to find him a wringer unit he couldn't possibly have sold. The television was newer, if only because TV sets hadn't been in existence all that long. This one was a twelve-inch Easy Vision Hoffman with a yellow screen—the failed concept of some promotion genius who had undoubtedly been fired long ago. Obviously his father had given all the appliances to Dana because they were cluttering up his warehouse and he didn't know what else to do with them.

Dana's father's actions were confusing to Ann. He seemed two-faced to her; she felt she could never be certain of what he was actually like. The "gift" of the appliances seemed cheap and almost cruel. Yet at the same time he had Dana and Ann join him, Brenda, and some of their friends in the finest clubs in town for parties costing as much as $400. He always paid the bill himself, with a flourish. In fact, some weeks it was not unusual for him to spend $1,000 on entertaining, and he usually invited Dana and Ann to be a part of it.

At first those evenings at supper clubs were exciting for Dana and Ann. They enjoyed the shows and the chance to eat food they couldn't afford on Dana's salary. But Brenda seemed to resent Ann and took every opportunity to make nasty remarks to her.

Ann became pregnant during that first year of marriage and was extremely happy about it. Dana was also pleased.

He felt that it was important for him to raise a child differently from the way his father had. He wanted to give the child all the love and attention he possibly could, to create an individual who would feel secure and wanted. He wanted to raise a child who would never know the trauma and loneliness he had known.

Now the apartment suddenly seemed small to Dana and Ann. They were considering a move when his father informed Dana that he had made arrangements with a realtor friend of his to get them a duplex near the city limits. Dana would be able to buy it with no down payment. His father would lie about Dana's income so that they would be certain to obtain financing. There was little chance of anybody's questioning the financial statement. All his father would have to do would be to say that Dana, the son of the owner and, by then, a top salesman, was earning at least as much as the average commissioned salesman working for the same firm—never mind that he was actually earning at least $75 a week less.

His father also stressed the investment value of the duplex. Monthly payments would be roughly $85, just about what they could charge to rent out the half of the duplex house they wouldn't be using.

Dana and Ann decided to take his father's advice. Both halves of the duplex were currently being rented, so the mortgage payments were of no consequence at the moment. One of the tenants would be moving out in a month, and the two and a half members of the Hawksworth family prepared to move into the vacant half.

During this period Johnny made occasional appearances, but even he had been subdued somewhat by married life. He tended to come out less often, and he caused Dana minimal trouble. Usually he would take over after Dana had left work to return home. He would go out drinking, not returning to Ann until three in the morning. Dana would have one excuse or another, none of which she believed. However, Ann loved him and found him attentive and kind most of the time, so she accepted his erratic behavior.

The only real embarrassment to her occurred a week before Ann and Dana were to move into the new duplex. A cleaning party had been planned at the new place. Ann's parents, brother, sister-in-law, and a couple of close friends all gathered to scrub the woodwork and generally get the place in shape.

When the housework was done, everyone sat around enjoying the beer, liquor, soft drinks, and food Dana had bought as a way of thanking them. There was much laughter and merriment, though Dana remained subdued as usual. His rather detached attitude was noticed by Ann's mother, who commented that it would be nice if he enjoyed himself more. "Why don't you come out of your shell, Dana, and join the fun?" she asked.

Dana was tired from the work and relaxed from the beer he had been drinking. As soon as Ann's mother made her comment, his eyes glazed over. A moment later Johnny was in the room.

"So you think there isn't enough excitement around here, do you?" he said, leering at everyone as he rose from his chair. Ann recognized the change in Dana immediately, though no one else realized what was happening.

Johnny stalked over to the phonograph, grabbed a record, and put it on the turntable. As the sounds of "The Hawaiian War Chant" came through the speaker, he began dancing wildly, leaping into the air, tossing back his head, howling insanely.

Soon he kicked off his shoes. Then he unbuttoned his shirt as everyone shouted at him. He threw the shirt to his "audience," then leaped into the air as he began unbuckling his pants.

The landing was not what he had expected. He hit the ground with his bare foot at an awkward angle. His arch bone snapped, the sound echoing through the room like a shot.

Pain leaped through the body. Johnny enjoyed the sufferings of others, but not his own. He immediately submerged, leaving Dana to face the agony of the injury and the humiliation of being half dressed in front of Ann's family.

Dana had to be taken to the hospital so the broken bone could be set in a cast. For the next six weeks he dragged about with him the heavy reminder of an incident he had no recollection of.

During that year Dana became the top salesman at the appliance store, moving more merchandise than any of the other eight salespeople. Since most of them were taking home $200 a week or more, and since Dana was selling more than any of them in addition to having management responsibilities, his father raised his pay—to $127.50 a week. He was forced to sell the Mercury and bought a very used 1950 Hudson for $250, which he had to borrow from a friend at $5 a week. He also had to pay the hospital in advance for the baby that was on the way, because his father refused to offer him medical insurance as an employee benefit.

Finally the nine months of pregnancy were over. "The pains are coming," said Ann happily. In anticipation, she had had her bag packed for several days.

Dana and Ann arrived at the hospital early in the morning. The pains were coming with increasing frequency but the baby was not about to make an early entrance into the world. By nine o'clock, it still had not been born.

"Ann's having the baby," said Dana, speaking excitedly to his father over the telephone. The appliance store had not opened for business yet.

"Has it been born?" asked his father.

"No. The doctor says it might not come till afternoon. I'm going to stay with her until it gets here."

"What the hell do you mean? You'd better get in to work," said his father angrily. "I'm not giving you a day off when the kid hasn't even come yet. You tell the hospital to call you at work whenever the baby actually arrives!"

"No," said Dana. "I can't do that. My place is with Ann. I'm going to stay here until the baby comes."

"If you want to be with Ann while business is going on,

that's fine with me. But you're going to have to start looking for another job. Unless you get over here at once,
you're fired! Do I make myself clear?"

Dana was deeply hurt by his father's attitude. His place
was with Ann, yet the couple had no money and he knew
that the threat of being fired was a serious one. Reluctantly he returned to the store.

At eleven o'clock the baby decided it wanted to be born
in time for lunch. The doctor called Dana to inform him
that he was the father of a healthy baby girl.

Dana dropped the telephone and rushed from the store.
He didn't bother to tell his father where he was going. All
that was on his mind was seeing Ann and the daughter,
Linda, whose name they had agreed on several weeks earlier.

But there was no great emotional reaction when Dana
saw his daughter for the first time. He felt no strong out-
pouring of love; he was incapable of such feelings. Peter
could have written reams of poetry about the birth had
Linda been his child, but Dana was incapable of such sen-
timent.

The one reaction he did have was a strong sense of obli-
gation to his daughter. He had helped bring the infant into
the world and he wanted to make her home life something
far different from what he had known growing up. His
daughter would know that her parents cared for her. He
would spend time with her and help her to grow into a
healthy, emotionally sound woman.

CHAPTER 14

As Linda began to grow, Dana took a keen interest in both her development and his own. He would frequently buy toys for her, selecting those that would provide a learning experience as well as being fun for her to play with. He wanted to nurture her mind so she might develop her full potential.

At the same time he was studying books on religion, mysticism, and the occult, hoping to find some clue to his own life. For the first time he had a reason to want to live like everyone else. The periods of amnesia he had been suffering put a strain on his home life and he was anxious to rid himself of them. He hoped the books might trigger some response in his mind; unfortunately, they failed to provide any answers.

In addition to his reading, he was also becoming increasingly sensitive to the way others lived. He recognized that many people exhibited extremes of emotion he knew nothing about. They always seemed to enjoy the good times more completely than he did and suffered the bad times with far more sensitivity. Even at home Ann commented that his approach to sex lacked the emotion that she felt. He read every sex manual he could find, hoping that a more sophisticated knowledge of lovemaking would give his wife the satisfaction she seemed to be missing. But such knowledge made sex no different from the way he handled life in general—mechanical and devoid of real feeling. He was saddened by his limitations and did not know how to correct them.

During this time his father's business prospered to the point where he decided to branch into a different but somewhat related line. He bought a building down the street from the appliance store, stocked it with new furniture, and put Dana in charge of it. He also gave Dana a raise to $135 a week.

There was still fairly good feeling between father and son even though Dana knew that he was being used. His father promised him a full partnership in the business one day, at which time there would be an even split of the profits. He was also heir to the business when his father decided to retire. So he looked upon himself as working for the future and accepted an income lower than almost anyone connected with the stores.

He was determined to make a success of himself. Since his only business background had come from on-the-job training he signed up for two correspondence courses—one in business management and another in interior decorating.

The training helped Dana in his selling, but it also made him aware of a new problem. His father, he discovered, was operating on a cash-flow basis; he had no money put away to cover expenses during bad times. Everything was based on people paying their bills as soon as they came due. The money went out as fast as it came in. If it should ever come in slower than anticipated, they would not have enough cash on hand to meet their own obligations. His father was drawing every cent of profit out of the store the moment it was taken in so he could continue his lavish spending.

Dana told his father about the problem, but his father refused to listen to him. He had built the business from nothing and considered himself a promotional genius. So long as the company was providing him with the money he wanted, he assumed he was doing everything right. It was to prove a disastrous mistake.

A second child was born to Dana and Ann three years after the first. Mark was their first son, and Dana delighted in the chance to raise him far differently from the way he had been reared.

But domestic life was rapidly paling for Johnny. One morning Dana was going to work later than usual. He didn't have to be at the store until noon since he would be staying late that night. He was on his way into town in the pickup truck he owned at the time, when Johnny took control of the wheel and headed for a bar in one of the rougher areas of the city.

Johnny swaggered into the bar, barely noticing the gang of motorcyclists drinking beer at a corner table. There were four of them, all tall and muscular with sleeveless shirts and tattoos on their arms. One bore the scars of a knife fight, while another had a slash mark where he had been struck by a chain. A third had folds of fat under his chin and wore dark glasses despite the fact that the bar was dimly lighted.

Johnny selected a stool and quickly downed two drinks. When he started to order his third, he realized he was out of money. "Can you cash a check?" he asked the bartender.

"If you're from around here and got some identification, I can," he said.

"Yeah, I got a local address," said Johnny.

"Okay. But no more than ten bucks."

Johnny wrote out the check, using Dana's pen. He showed the bartender his identification and was given the money. The bartender put the check in the cash register, then picked up the pen, apparently thinking it was his own.

"What the hell you doing with my pen, buddy?" said Johnny.

"Sorry, fella, but that's not your pen. It belongs to the bar."

"Give me back that fuckin' pen!"

"Smartass troublemakers I can do without," said the bartender. "You've had your drinks. Go on home."

In the corner of the room the four gang members stopped talking and looked over at the bar. They were friends of the bartender and they tensed for trouble. If Johnny didn't leave on his own, they were obviously thinking, they'd bounce his ass into the street. But Johnny ignored them.

He reached over the bar, grabbing the bartender by the collar and pulling him completely over the top of the bar, then hurling him to the floor. The four gang members pushed back their chairs, knocking their table over as they moved towards Johnny.

Johnny turned, grabbed a bar stool, and slammed it into them, scattering them across the floor. One of the gang started to rise, but as he gained his feet Johnny kicked him in the chin, knocking him cold. Then he picked up a second stool and threw it at the others.

Meanwhile another patron slipped out to call the police. In moments two officers came running into the bar.

Johnny grabbed a third stool and ran at the officers. They tried to duck out of the way but were struck down.

As Johnny went out the door he almost collided with another officer. The policeman grabbed him and got him in an arm lock—but Johnny wrestled his way free, slamming his elbow into the officer's stomach.

The two policemen in the bar, meanwhile, had come back out, and the three of them finally overcame Johnny. He was handcuffed, thrown into the squad car, and taken off to jail.

He actually enjoyed the ride. There was no place to keep him locally so he had to be driven thirty miles to the county holding facility. Along the way he laughed at the officers, cursed them, and had a thoroughly good time.

When they arrived at the jail all his possessions were

removed for safekeeping. He had only a few dollars with him but he decided to get the arresting officers in trouble. "Hey," he shouted after he had emptied his wallet. "These sons-of-bitches stole a hundred-dollar bill from me. I had it when they arrested me and it's gone now. You can't trust anybody. Make the bastards give me back my money!"

The jailer was stunned by Johnny's outburst.

"I saw them steal it! When they put the handcuffs on me they pulled the $100 out of my pocket. Hell, they're a bunch of crooks! I want you to put *that* down on the paper!" He pointed at the property slip—an itemized list of all a prisoner's possessions at the time he entered jail. Persons under arrest were told to sign it after everything had been removed from their pockets. Upon their release all the items that had been listed were returned to them. Johnny insisted they add the $100 bill he had never had but which he claimed had been stolen from him.

"I won't sign anything until my complaint is put in writing. If you bastards try to charge me with anything, I'm going to charge those sons-of-bitches with stealing my money!"

The jailer didn't believe Johnny but he wasn't going to argue with him. He wrote down that Johnny claimed he had had a hundred-dollar bill at the time of his arrest but that there was no sign of it when his possessions were itemized. Then he put Johnny into a single holding cell rather than the drunk tank because he felt he was likely to harm the other prisoners.

Johnny amused himself in the cell by shouting obscenities at everyone. Then gradually he became bored, and finally he submerged. Phil took control.

He called the jailer to the cell. Polite, even-tempered, and calm, he apologized for Johnny's action and asked if he could make a telephone call.

The jailer was startled at how quickly Johnny had sobered up and changed his attitude, not realizing that he was speaking to a different personality. He let him phone Ann, who agreed to raise the $150 bail.

Phil allowed Dana to resume control after Ann arrived
to free him. When Dana, shocked to find himself in jail,
asked what had happened, he was shown the charges
against him. His last memory was of being on his way to
work, but he lied and said he had stopped for a drink because he was concerned about business pressures. Ann
would worry about his drinking so early in the day, he
knew, but he simply couldn't offer more of an explanation.

At Dana's court appearance three days later, the judge
read the report of his crimes, stopping occasionally to look
at him. The judge's face wore a broad grin and he broke
into laughter periodically. Apparently the barroom brawl
described in the police report reminded him of an old John
Wayne movie. Rather than being concerned about Dana's
state of mind or potential for violence in the future, he
took the entire incident as a joke.

"How do you plead?" asked the judge when he had finished reading.

"I plead guilty, your honor," said Dana, ashamed of himself.

"Well, I'm going to let you off easy," said the judge, grinning broadly. "I'll charge you a $50 fine and put you on a
year's probation. Now, you don't have to report to a probation officer during the next year. However, I'm going to
insist. . . . " the judge started to laugh. "I'm going to insist
that during that year you don't watch any more westerns
on television."

Dana's erratic behavior during this time had an effect
on his social life as well. His father stopped inviting him to
his parties and evenings on the town. Dana didn't drink if
he stayed himself, and his father didn't like to be in the
company of someone who didn't enjoy booze. Yet when
Dana became Johnny, the pleasures of his drinking companionship were ruined by his sudden tendency to tell his
father exactly what he thought of him. If his father refused to listen to his abuse, Johnny would start a brawl
simply to embarrass him.

Ann had made a number of personal friends, but she
and Dana could never spend time with them as a couple.

She was embarrassed by his changes in behavior and did not want to take the chance of her friends unexpectedly meeting Johnny or Peter. So she took to visiting her friends alone. She didn't enjoy that, either, but Dana had become too unpredictable. She only risked going out with him when they were visiting her family; they accepted him even without understanding his actions.

The beginning of the end of Dana's career at his father's store came when Brenda decided one day to take an active part in the business. She was interested in fashions and had talked with several representatives of clothing manufacturers who specialized in expensive children's wear. There were no shops carrying such clothing in the entire community, and she learned she could acquire exclusive rights to sell it, as well as quality toys, children's furniture, and related items. She felt that if the furniture store were closed, the space it occupied could be used to put in the items she wanted, which she would then sell herself.

There were several things wrong with this plan. The first was that she had no experience in this type of retailing, nor did Dana or his father. Marketing clothing required an entirely different approach from marketing "large-ticket" items such as those Dana and his father had been selling successfully for years. She assumed, however, that if one business could be successful with the Hawksworth name, a totally unrelated business could also make money.

Another problem was that she wanted to close the furniture store even though it was making a steady profit. Things might not have been so bad if she had opened her business in another location, but closing down a money-making operation to start something new seemed illogical, to say the least.

But logic meant nothing to Dana's father and Brenda. They were convinced that anything they tried to sell would make them money; they weren't about to listen to Dana's objections. The furniture store would close and Dana would return to work in the appliance division.

What neither Dana nor his father suspected was that the

one store would not be enough for Brenda. She had a friend who ran a large discount house. She had secretly arranged with him to lease a section of his store so she could put her expensive line of children's items there as well. The fact that people shopping in a discount house have little interest in buying premium goods never crossed her mind. And her friend didn't caution her about it because he made his money when he leased her the space; he wanted her as a tenant.

His father brought Dana back to the appliance store as general manager and gave him a raise to $140 a week. Even at that he was almost the lowest-paid employee in the place, but he still believed he was working for the future. One day everything would be his.

The new clothing operation started out losing money and went downhill from there. Brenda knew nothing about stocking and moving the merchandise. When the seasons changed, she was left with a huge inventory of undesirable merchandise, which she had to sell below cost just to clear it out. She kept pleading that all she needed was time. The business would be a success if Dana's father would just be patient a little while longer.

Soon he was pulling every spare dollar he could from the appliance business and giving it to Brenda for her clothing store. He even went so far as to break the law for her. The appliance store's inventory was owned by the bank. When the merchandise was sold, the bank was paid off and the difference between the selling price and the bank loan paid for overhead and profit. By juggling the books, Dana's father was able to delay paying the bank for merchandise that had already been sold. That "spare" capital went to Brenda.

Then one day one of the bank examiners became suspicious, probably because, according to his records, Dana's father was suddenly selling less than he had been in the past. A surprise check was made; Dana's father could not account for $63,000.

That year—1959—the appliance store had had gross

sales in excess of $1,000,000, with a net profit in excess of $75,000. Yet because of Dana's father plunging the money into Brenda's business, it had gone broke!

There were immediate threats of criminal action. Dana was determined to save the business if at all possible. He knew that if he and his father could return the money owed to the bank, they might still be able to survive. He began working sixteen-hour days, cutting costs to the bone and handling as many tasks himself as he possibly could to save on employee salaries.

His father, however, couldn't adjust to the realities of failure. He had gambled on the woman he loved and lost everything; moreover, he was overwhelmed by the thought that he might have to abandon his old life style. Instead of pitching in to help Dana save the business, he took to drinking and playing cards every day with the Mafia don he knew and some of their friends. Dana drew no salary. Instead, when his father won at cards he would be given $100 or $200 to meet his personal expenses. When his father lost, he would have to pull money from the business to cover the amount.

Meanwhile Brenda kept insisting that she would make it, and Dana's father continued to give her everything she wanted. He refused to let Dana have any control over the checkbook, so money kept going out while the business went downhill.

Soon Dana's father was spending as much as $1,000 a week on drinking, gambling, and entertaining. It was almost as though he thought that if he ignored the realities of his economic situation, everything would be all right.

Finally Dana recruited and trained a crew of seven salesmen to go door-to-door in a section of the city that housed families of Navy men stationed at a nearby base. They were to sell high-profit items to bring in a surge of new money. The salesmen were successful and considerable sums were brought in, but not nearly enough to offset his father's free-spending life style.

Dana gradually managed to pay off the $63,000 owed the

bank and arranged for over $100,000 in credit from merchandisers so the store's stock could be replenished. He had to assure the merchandisers that he was going to have a stronger hand in the business and that his father would limit himself to the promotional aspects for which he had earned everyone's respect. He hoped in this way that they could survive until November, the start of their big selling season, a period that could put them back on their feet.

Dana stressed to his father that he would have to stop taking money from the business for his personal use. He told Brenda that if she sold only the merchandise she already had on hand and didn't try to replenish it with funds from the appliance store, they just might survive. Neither listened to him.

As the end of the business came near, Dana was working alone one Sunday, handling all sales and clerical work himself to save overhead. His father came in for the first time in a week and said he wanted a couple of blank checks. "Brenda and I have been quite tense about business problems," he said. "We think what we need is to get away from everything for a few days. We're going to go to Las Vegas to do a little gambling."

The news churned Dana's stomach. His father and Brenda had never spent less than $10,000 on any of their Las Vegas trips. If they took blank checks—and there was no way Dana could stop them—all his hard work would be for nothing. He tried to argue, but it was no use. His father took what he wanted and left.

"To hell with it," thought Dana. "To hell with every Goddamned thing!" He called Ann to tell her he was closing the store and coming home.

He had never felt so hurt and angry. He wanted to explode, yet his emotions remained controlled—as they always did. He got into his car, turned the ignition, and Johnny took over.

Johnny could handle the hatred Dana was incapable of feeling. He cursed as he drove, then pulled into a bar and began drinking heavily. He decided to have a little fun himself and headed for the state line, getting stopped along the way for speeding and drunken driving. He spent the night in jail and Dana took over the next morning. In court that day, Dana was found guilty on all counts, including assault on a police officer, and was given twenty-eight days in jail. Two weeks into his sentence his father's business was finally padlocked and closed for good.

CHAPTER 15

The failure of his father's business marked the end of financial stability for Dana—or at least the end of whatever job security his father's business had been able to provide, no matter how poor the financial benefits had been. In the years to come, he would find and quickly lose a rapid succession of jobs in a variety of fields—his proven executive ability assuring his finding ready employment, and his constant blackouts assuring that he would not be able to hold it for long.

As a direct result of the business failure, Dana was forced into bankruptcy. He lost his house and most of his other possessions. He also had to handle the onslaught of creditors who had dealt with his father. In the end his father also had to declare bankruptcy. He lost his two Cadillacs, his mansion, and his boat.

Eventually his father became a salesman for a furniture store, quickly becoming their number-one man. However, his income was only $1,000 a month, so Brenda also had to go to work as well. She passed the examination to get a real estate license and found a job with a realtor.

Dana went to work at an appliance store and immediately did well there. With the commissions he earned, his income was more than it had been when he had worked for his father. Ann took a job as a solderer for Western Electric to bring in extra money, since certain of their debts had not been wiped out by the bankruptcy.

During this period Dana owned a large German Shepherd. It adored Ann and the children but was totally devoted to Dana, spending most of his time by his master's side whenever Dana was at home. It didn't matter whether he arrived at noon or two in the morning, the dog knew the sound of his car and would happily rush to see him, licking him and wagging his tail eagerly.

Johnny was afraid of dogs and didn't like the idea of being around the Shepherd. He made certain he was gone when the dog was around. He let Dana resume control whenever he was returning home if he thought the dog might be running loose.

But Johnny had been drinking that New Year's Eve so he wasn't thinking as clearly as usual. He was determined to stay in control and try to have sex with Ann even though she always rejected what she considered Dana's "Mr. Hyde" aspect. As he pulled the car into the garage he thought of the dog, then dismissed the animal as being of no consequence.

"Hell, I look enough like the chickenshit to fool that damn mutt. He'll think I'm Dana and I won't have to worry about him." He opened the door and stepped inside the house.

The dog was upstairs when the car pulled into the garage but his sensitive hearing picked up the familiar sound. His tail began wagging and he bounded happily to the top of the stairs, expecting to see Dana.

Johnny glanced up at the dog and began to walk up the stairs. "It's me, your master, you stupid mutt," he mumbled.

The dog tensed, knowing that whoever was approaching him *wasn't* his master and that he wasn't going to let him endanger his home and the humans he loved. A low growl came to his throat as he started slowly down the steps. He paused, studied the man who was coming closer, then leaped at Johnny, knocking him to the ground. He bared his teeth and moved in towards Johnny's throat.

Johnny, frightened half out of his wits, immediately submerged, leaving a bewildered Dana in control.

The dog had been ready to kill an instant before. Now his head jerked back and his tail dropped between his legs. The growl turned to a cry of anguish. He had been about to tear out the throat of the person he loved most, a person he was certain had not been there earlier. Confused and frightened, he moved to a corner of the room, his body shaking. It was several hours before he calmed down.

A short while later Ann gave birth to another son, Scott. Dana was as devoted to him as he was to his other children. His efforts to help them grow up happily would stay in Ann's mind later, whenever she considered leaving him after a Johnny or Peter incident. The good times always outweighed the bad in her mind.

And soon Dana was changing jobs and homes on a regular basis. He also was frequently in court for assault and battery, drunk driving charges, and related offenses—gifts to him left behind by an unrepentant Johnny.

Periodically Dana and Ann had trial separations. Dana would go to a hotel to live for a few days while Ann stayed in the house. During these periods Peter would often write poetry throughout the night. Some of it interested Dana a great deal when he found it in the morning, although he had no idea where it had come from.

"Bridges" was the title of one such poem:

> Caissons clunk 'cross wooden floors
> Mighty rivers rage 'round concrete piles
>   Its thunderous voice
>   Muted by the while of black rubber
>   Hurtling people going and coming
> A wee brook tinkles below

Aged-warped oak A
Magpie perched on
        The rotten wood rail
Sings its song
Miles of steel and concrete
    Span the vast ocean bays
    bringing together great cities
            While strange ships
            From distant ports pass beneath
And somewhere
        There is a new bridge
        Cradling brave soldiers
                going to battle
Passing dead comrades
        Going home Forever

Another was titled, simply, "Love's Gift":

Lovers apart unknowing of the other,
Each one yearning for that magic meeting
That brings together the father and mother
Of life yet unborn and love completing,
Often by way of pain, its only goal.
The miraculous double creation
Of new life and two spirits into one soul
Locked in time without termination.
Incomplete is a woman or a man
Wandering in the search for love's gift
Of wholeness, as promised before life began,
When the spirit craved, that was once adrift,
To be merged with another and become one,
Letting Love triumph and its miracle be done.

Dana himself began studying religion, philosophy, and
any other field he thought might give him some answers
about himself. But there seemed to be no logical explanation for what others claimed was his extremely bizarre
behavior during those periods when he suffered blackouts.

Perhaps, he thought, everyone was simply exaggerating; perhaps there was nothing at all wrong with him. He decided all he needed was a strong act of will to keep himself under control. Yet such personal determination was never enough to prevent Johnny, Peter, and Phil from manipulating his actions.

Perhaps the most troublesome time for Dana came when he got a job with the Leonard Cohn Furniture Store. It was run by Rachel Cohn and her son, Leonard Junior.

The furniture store was a small family operation with Dana the only salesman, besides the Cohns, on the floor. He was successful from the start and immediately got along well with the Cohns, who respected his abilities as a salesman.

The family had an interesting history. The late owner had for years been a major financial power in the community. He had extensive land holdings and was engaged in numerous business deals. Unfortunately he could not cope with his high-pressure life style, and in time became an alcoholic. His mind and body quickly deteriorated and his associates swindled him out of his multimillion-dollar fortune. The family was left without funds.

Leonard Junior decided to bail his father out of trouble. He started a furniture store and worked to pay his father's debts and restore the family fortune. His mother was put in charge of the used furniture department. Her salary arrangement was rather unusual. Officially she was paid $500 a month; unofficially her son let her pocket the down payments on any furniture she sold, then write up the orders on a net basis. That way she supplemented her income without having to report it on her tax return.

The Cohns were extremely sensitive about their Jewish religion. The father's partners had been Gentiles and the family was quite bitter about the way they had taken advantage of him. Dana was the first Gentile they had ever considered hiring for their store, thereby extending a trust to him that they had never shown anyone else. Mrs. Cohn, during slow business hours, would even talk to Dana about the history and culture of the Jewish people so he would have more of an understanding of them and their ways.

Less than two months after Dana began working at the furniture store, Johnny took control one day during his lunch break. He went to a bar for a few drinks, then decided to raise some hell at the store and see if he could get Dana fired.

Johnny had never been a biased individual in the way most people think of prejudice. He did not have a special hatred for any particular person or group of people. He didn't care if someone was white, black, Jew, Gentile, Moslem, or whatever. He hated everyone equally.

So when he walked into the furniture store that day and went to see Leonard, what came out could hardly have been more surprising. "You stinking New York kike," said Johnny. "When I look at slime like you I know Hitler was right.

"You're a nothing; a zero! Your kike father couldn't hold onto his money. He was a sot—a stinking Jew sot rotting in a garbage pit.

"And your mother's no better. She's been worthless for years. She's a leech and a has-been."

The tirade continued, the language crude and the tone extremely bitter.

Leonard Cohn was normally an explosive man, a person who managed to keep his temper just barely under control during the best of times. But he did not get violent when he heard Johnny speak. Instead he was crushed. His shoulders sagged and his head bowed. He had trusted Dana. He had grown to look upon him almost as a brother. He had opened his heart to this Gentile and thought that at last he had found a man of another religion who could empathize with him. The words completely shattered him.

When Johnny realized Leonard wasn't going to strike him, he thought it was the funniest thing he had seen in years. He began laughing uncontrollably and walked out of the store, knowing that Dana was through in that job.

But the initial shock of Johnny's tirade wore off quickly.

Leonard was convinced there was something wrong. He couldn't believe the man who had just spoken so cruelly to him was the same person he had gotten to know over the past few weeks. He decided to call Ann and ask whether something had been troubling Dana that day.

Ann was upset by the telephone call. She knew this side of her husband's personality, but what could she tell Leonard? She didn't want to jeopardize her husband's job. Finally she said that Dana had an occasional drinking problem, which was apparently related to the trauma of his father's business failures. If Leonard would only be patient with him, she added, she was certain Dana would get control of it.

Leonard believed the story because he wanted to believe it. He had been hurt by those he trusted in the past and he didn't want to be hurt again. It was easier for him to continue working with Dana than to admit he had been fooled by the man.

Dana returned the following day, his only knowledge of the incident coming from what others had told him. He was sickened by what little he heard. He knew the outburst, if it had really occurred, in no way reflected his personal feelings for Leonard Cohn. Yet the reception he received from Leonard was guarded; Dana knew something quite serious must have happened.

Leonard told Dana that he felt every Gentile, deep down inside, had anti-Semitic feelings. He said that the drinking Dana had done on his lunch hour probably had brought this hidden anti-Semitism to the surface. He was sorry that the feelings existed in Dana but he would spend as much time as he could explaining about Jewish people so Dana could overcome the bias.

Leonard's attempt to understand Dana was deeply moving, yet Dana knew he had no anti-Semitic feelings. He had a great respect for the Jewish people and what they had overcome to achieve success in American society. Even if he hadn't, he was incapable of such extremes of emotion as Leonard said he had shown the day before. Yet he did not argue with Leonard. He liked his employer and wanted to retain his job.

During the next few weeks the two of them grew even closer than they had been before the Johnny incident. Their families ate at each other's homes and Dana was invited to one of Leonard's poker parties. Leonard wanted to make Dana a part of his personal as well as his business life.

Dana's limited emotional range prevented him from fully appreciating what Leonard was trying to do. Despite Johnny's best efforts, Leonard was reaching out to him in the true spirit of friendship. He became as close to Dana as Noel had been. This inability to give or receive the total love of which a normal person is capable was the curse and the tragedy of Dana's existence. He recognized the fact, but could do nothing about it.

The months passed quickly and business increased at a steady rate. Leonard put more money into advertising to bring people into the store, and Dana's sales ability ensured that most of those who entered stayed to buy. Soon Leonard asked Dana to hire a part-time salesman to work nights and weekends so Dana could have some time off. He would receive an override on the salesman's volume so his own income would not be hurt. For the first time in months Dana was able to work less than a six-day week and could spend weekends with his family. It was a luxury he thoroughly enjoyed.

Several months passed before Johnny came in control once more in a way that hurt Dana. Johnny had gotten drunk, then gone on a wild 100-mile-an-hour ride pursued by police, sheriff's deputies, and highway patrolmen. As a result, Dana's license was revoked for three years and he was given a thirty-day jail sentence.

Leonard provided a lawyer for Dana and worked to get the jail sentence suspended. Ann, who had been at the trial, also talked with the judge, and their combined pleas worked in Dana's favor. The jail term was suspended, but Dana would not be allowed to drive.

Once again Dana and Ann had to move, this time into a house Leonard sold them. It was close enough to work so that Dana's lack of a driver's license would not be a problem. Leonard arranged to move their possessions and didn't even charge them a down payment.

In addition to his furniture business, Leonard had a real estate license, and he began to take an increasingly active interest in the real estate field. Several weeks after the trial he told Dana that in the near future the furniture store would be closed. When changes were made in the business, he added, they would happen very quickly; Dana should be prepared. He suggested that he begin looking around for another job.

Two weeks later, the furniture warehouse was suddenly burglarized and most of the carpeting stored there was stolen. Dana didn't believe any thief could have taken the carpeting; it was in the form of five 1,000-pound rolls, which could not be moved without special equipment. He suspected that Leonard had arranged the theft himself, and that he had probably used or sold the carpeting, then decided to collect an insurance payment on it as well. However, neither the police nor the insurance investigators could prove that it hadn't been stolen.

Two weeks after that Dana was shocked one morning to discover that the store had burned to the ground during the night. The police immediately suspected arson, but once more were unable to come up with clear proof. The insurance investigators were equally suspicious. But the fire, if it had been the result of arson, had been set professionally, and there was simply no way that Leonard could be connected to it. The insurance company was forced to pay off.

Leonard immediately went full time into the real estate business, eventually becoming a major property owner in the area and wealthier than his father had been at his peak. Dana was given $750 severance pay to help tide him over until he could find a new job.

Two weeks later he found work at another furniture

store. He had to drive to get there but decided it was worth the risk. He couldn't let his family go hungry and there wasn't a way to take public transportation to the store's location.

That second job lasted only thirty days before a freak fire occurred and that store, too, burned to the ground.

Dana was numb from the twin fires, even though their occurrence, he was sure, was pure coincidence. He began to feel that if he worked in another furniture store and it, too, caught fire, the police might begin to suspect *him* of arson. It was time to go into a different business.

The year by now was 1961, and Dana's next job was one of the best he was ever to hold. He was hired by Conglomerate Underwriters Insurance Corporation as a salesman. His starting pay was just $550 a month, but he would not remain at that level for long.

Dana quickly grew to love the insurance business. He liked helping people plan their estates; they, in turn, appreciated his expertise in the field. He began selling more and more insurance and quickly joined the elite in the business by selling more than a million dollars in coverage in a single year.

Dana's combination of management expertise, success in selling, and knowledge of the field greatly impressed his bosses. He moved up quickly and by 1964 was the district manager for the company at a salary of $3,000 a month. He and his wife thought their financial problems at last were over.

Johnny and Peter had not been silent during these three years. From time to time Dana would be on his way to see a client or traveling home from work when the familiar depression would strike and he would black out for a few hours. When he again began to function, he would either be ill from a hangover or surrounded by reams of poems and essays. But the difference between an insurance salesman's life and the life of men in other fields is that everyone expects the salesman to keep unusual hours. Dana's disappearances may have inconvenienced a client occasion-

ally, but the absences were scarcely noticed by his employ-
ers. A little fast talking usually soothed his clients' feelings. Certainly he lost some business, but his overall
earnings were so high that no one noticed.

The management promotion, however, was the beginning of the end for that career, too. Dana was suddenly
responsible for all underwriting or direct marketing activities in his district—an area with a population of roughly
300,000. Each such district had an office where from four
to twenty-five agents were employed, in addition to secretaries and other personnel. There were fifteen agents directly responsible to Dana.

The offices themselves were impressive. They occupied
the entire third floor of a four-story building owned by the
insurance company. When you got off the elevator, you
walked down a short hall toward a large door with a sign
reading "Hawksworth District Conglomerate Underwriters Insurance Company—Dana Hawksworth District
Manager." Inside was a receptionist and beyond her a
large open area containing the desks of the newer agents.
Along one side ran a row of private offices for the more
experienced agents. The office farthest to the left was for
Dana's private secretary; his own office, a much larger
room, was behind hers.

Dana had been district manager for four months when
Johnny decided he was sick of Dana enjoying the good life.
Johnny's only pleasure came from the misery of others—
especially that goody-goody S.O.B. who was then a big
executive.

He took over the body sometime early in the morning
when Dana was not expecting trouble, and immediately
decided to get a few kicks by knocking Dana's reputation
down a few notches. He drove to the Conglomerate Underwriters building and parked in Dana's reserved space
in the first-floor garage.

"Good morning, Mr. Hawksworth," said an attractive secretary who passed him on the way to the elevator.

Johnny grabbed at her buttocks, sending her rushing

down the hall in confusion. She had had physical passes made at her before, but not by the normally staid district manager.

The elevator took Johnny to the third floor. He was impressed by the company offices. Dana was one hell of a big man—lord high chickenshit! Well, he would change all that.

"Good morning, Mr. Hawksworth," said the receptionist.

"Get your ass out of this office or I'll rape you where you're sitting," he said to her coldly. The secretary's mouth opened and she stared at him, stunned. Then she rose from her seat and fled out the door.

He continued to the rear of the room, where one of the secretaries was sharpening a pencil. She was better looking than the receptionist so he decided to have a little fun with her. "Take off your clothes," he said.

The secretary started to laugh. Dana Hawksworth was nice enough, but he was so reserved she often wondered how he was able to satisfy his wife. He certainly wasn't the type to make a sexual pass except as some sort of practical joke.

"I said take off your clothes," Johnny repeated, his low voice menacing. He grabbed her blouse, ripping it down the front and exposing her bra.

The secretary screamed and ran from the room, on the verge of hysteria, clutching her torn clothing. Johnny watched her run, laughing.

This place is too damned plush for that chickenshit Dana, he said to himself as he looked around at the expensive desks and thick carpeting on the floor of the District Manager's private office. He began walking from office to office, kicking open the doors and tossing over the desks. He was going to wreck the place.

"Mr. Hawksworth, have you gone mad?" asked one of the insurance agents. The agent was an elderly man who could have retired years earlier. He no longer did any selling, but came to the office every day merely to service his old clients.

Johnny turned toward the old man and hit him savagely

on the jaw. The blow could have flattened a much younger man. The agent slumped to the ground, barely conscious.

A second insurance agent went after Johnny. He was a youthful former police officer, still as trim and athletic as the day he quit the force. But even he was no match. Johnny grabbed a large, heavy desk, rushed towards the agent and slammed it into his stomach, doubling him over it as he crashed it into the wall. The agent was wedged solidly behind the desk, in great pain and gasping for breath. It was only by chance that his back hadn't been broken from the impact.

Johnny paused. The desks were all overturned and the doors broken, the office was in shambles. The rage he had felt upon entering was dissipating, but he wanted to do one last thing before leaving. He took a paperweight from the floor and heaved it through one of the glass windows.

Then, without another word, he left the building. The police had been called but had not yet arrived. He climbed into Dana's car and headed for a bar. He felt he had earned himself a drink.

The tremendous respect Dana had once commanded in the company was obvious from the way Conglomerate Underwriters handled the incident. Although both the agents Johnny had struck required medical attention, neither was seriously hurt. There was also relatively little furniture that had been broken beyond repair. Dana's superiors, therefore, decided they would refrain from filing criminal charges. Nor would they force Dana to pay for the damage Johnny had done. They did, however, fire him.

It would not be the last job he would lose because of Johnny's unpredictable activities. This one, however, proved to be particularly discouraging, for Ann as well as for himself. They had thought that, at last, things were going to be a little better for them. They had liked the life the job had offered, as well as the people it had brought them into contact with. They had begun to see some kind of a normal existence for them stretching out ahead.

And now, once more, they were back at the beginning, starting all over again.

CHAPTER **16**

It was during Dana's first year with the insurance agency that the possibility first occurred to him that his problems might be the result of alcoholism. His driving record by this time, of course, was peppered with drunken driving citations—virtually all of them picked up by Johnny during his periodic binges. The list of arrests, in fact, had seriously threatened for a time to block his license as an insurance agent. The possibility seemed a logical one—one at least that merited some checking out.

The idea that he might be an alcoholic actually pleased Dana to a degree. It would at least account for the blackouts he had suffered from and the unusual behavior he had exhibited during them. This explanation, of course, completely overlooked the fact that he had been experiencing periodic amnesia since shortly after his third birthday, but that didn't really matter to him. He liked the idea of being able to put a label on his erratic condition. He promptly joined Alcoholics Anonymous.

The time spent with this organization proved to be en-

joyable for both Dana and Ann. They liked the members of
the group to which he belonged and they made many
friends. However, as Dana listened to their stories, he began to suspect that his problems were probably not al-
cohol-related, even though he was frequently drinking during the periods about which he had no memory. He was,
he knew, very different from the other members who professed to be alcoholics.

He had been in AA about a year and a half when
Johnny finally grew sick of listening to the do-gooders put
down booze. He took control shortly before one of the meetings, went to a bar, and downed several drinks. Then he
went stomping into the meeting room, sauntered to the
front, and looked coldly at the assembled group. His eyes
narrowed as he leaned on the lectern and said, "My name
is Dana and I'm the only real alcoholic here. The rest of
you are drinking failures!"

Johnny opened his coat and pulled out two bottles of
whiskey and a half dozen glasses and placed them on a
table. As the members stared in amazement, he turned
and tromped out of the meeting room, laughing. He took a
plane to Reno and stayed there for a week.

Dana awakened in a hotel room feeling hung over. He
had no idea where he was or how much time had passed.
He made his way groggily into the bathroom, where he
saw a woman's panties and bra as well as some cosmetics
on the counter. He didn't know whose they were or when
the woman might come back.

Dana dressed quickly, then called Ann to tell her he
would be flying home. He had learned he was in Reno by
reading the room service menu on the table. He had plenty
of money in his wallet, something unusual for him after
one of these spells. He assumed that he had gambled successfully. It was little consolation.

Shortly after the Reno episode, Brenda added a new
complication to Dana's life by developing terminal cancer,
which began to affect her brain. Soon she was unable to
coordinate thought and speech. She would think one thing
and say something else.

Dana began visiting her every day. He felt sorry for her and they developed a kinship stronger than any they had ever known. He was the only person able to make sense of her confusing conversations and this made her happy to see him.

Brenda was a fighter to the end. She managed to survive for several months even though the doctors had given her a maximum of a few weeks to live. Dana admired her courage and the way she had stayed with his father through bad times as well as good. He was surprised to find himself genuinely saddened when she died.

Perhaps what touched him most about Brenda's last days was her changed attitude toward Ann. She expressed her respect for Ann's strength and love as a mother and asked her to keep an eye on Dana's half sister, who was nine at the time. She did not feel Dana's father could care properly for the child by himself and wanted to be certain Ann would make her welcome, providing guidance when possible. It saddened Dana that the two women couldn't have been reconciled earlier.

Dana's father was overwhelmed by grief for almost a week after the death. He moved in with Dana, leaning on him as he had when his first wife died. By the end of the week he felt strong enough to return home. Three days after that his mourning period apparently came to an end. He began living with another woman, the first of many such affairs he would enter into during the rest of his life.

And shortly after that Dana and Ann were struck by another tragedy. Their daughter Linda came down with rheumatic fever, a disease that can cause severe heart damage and often cripples those who get it. For nine months she remained almost immobile. Her education was handled by a tutor, though her weakened condition made studying difficult.

Then, after following an intense drug treatment program, she was restored to health. Her body had been weakened but not seriously damaged. More important, she was left with an overwhelming drive to excel, both mentally and physically.

Linda was put back a half year in school but soon became top in her class. Before the illness she had been satisfied with passing grades. She also became an athlete, participating in track and field and related sports requiring great physical exertion. She set school, county, and state records, many of which have not been broken to this day. Her achievements delighted Dana. The love he could feel for all his children, limited though it was, made him want to overcome his own problems and be more like the fathers of other children.

After Johnny wrecked the insurance company office, Dana went to work for another insurance company more than an hour's drive from his home. The commuting time proved to be too much for him and he left that job after only three weeks. However, while he was there he met Steve Shaw, a successful Certified Life Underwriter, one of the elite in the profession. This meeting resulted in another job that would prove to be a highlight of Dana's professional life.

Steve Shaw, a wealthy man, was a law school graduate as well as C. L. U. He had plans to open a corporation that would be a combined insurance, trust, and mortgage company. After learning of Dana's marketing expertise, he asked him to become executive vice-president for a high salary and ten percent of the stock in the new business.

Dana was enthusiastic about the opportunity. He immediately enrolled in an accelerated real estate school to complete his knowledge in the fields the firm would be handling. He already understood marketing and insurance.

The corporation leased a suite of offices, using money from a life insurance company that was backing the venture. Dana was given a $2,000-a-month corporate salary as well as commissions on business he handled and bonuses based on profit. He planned a marketing program that would reach the young executive on the rise—the man or woman in the $20,000-to-$25,000 bracket who promised to move still higher in his firm. The competitors in the field waited until someone actually achieved a high bracket before going after his or her business. Dana felt that if his new company could get the business earlier, they would be able to retain it even after the rising executive reached the top.

The corporation handled estate planning, the establishment of trusts in its own trust company, refinancing of real estate holdings to free cash for investing, and similar matters.

The idea was immediately successful. Dana was heading a multimillion-dollar business within six months. He had quickly added thirty-two salesmen, three sales supervisors, and a sales manager to the staff. He also began studying law through an extension program.

He was also in the unusual position of being his own father's superior. His father, some time before, had entered the insurance business himself, and Dana soon hired him as a sales supervisor in the new firm. Despite the ill will that had existed between them, he recognized his father's tremendous promotion and sales abilities and felt he would be an asset in the firm.

Dana and Ann moved into an expensive home, and he became a Sunday School teacher for a wealthy Presbyterian Church in the area. He came to be respected by everyone.

But once the organization was functioning well enough on its own so Dana didn't have to constantly oversee all activities, Johnny found he could come out at will. Dana only had to be in the office in the morning to give the day's instructions to his secretary. After that, he didn't have to account for his time to anyone.

Many of the Johnny takeovers were short-term. Half way through the day he might take control and spend the rest of the afternoon drinking.

Perhaps the most bizarre incident during this period took place on a trip to Los Angeles. Dana and his key executives were attending a special training program to learn how to interview potential executive and sales employees.

Dana had planned to be in Los Angeles during the first

day of the session only. He felt he did not need the specialized training, due to the nature of his particular position. However, he had been asked to give the opening speech at a major hotel in Burbank.

The day went quite well. The response to the speech was enthusiastic and Dana enjoyed the rest of the morning session. He ate with the men, observed the afternoon class, and then made plans to fly home that evening following a dinner arranged by the insurance company that was underwriting his corporation.

One of the supervisors, Art Blackman, had rented a car to use during his stay in Los Angeles. After dinner Dana asked Art if he would drive him to the airport so he could catch his 7:30 plane. Naturally Art wouldn't say no to his boss, so the two of them went to the airport, arriving early.

"Let me buy you a drink while we're waiting for your plane to start boarding," said Art.

"I don't really want anything to drink, but you go ahead and I'll have a Coke to keep you company," said Dana. The two men went to one of the airport cocktail lounges and took two stools at the bar.

Dana sipped his Coke, talking with Art about the events of the day. Suddenly he felt strange, almost as if he were developing the flu. "I don't feel well," he said, closing his eyes. His face became strained.

"What's the matter, Dana?" asked Art, concerned. But Dana was no longer there. A wave of depression had followed the sick feeling and Johnny had taken over.

"Matter?" said Johnny. "Shit, I never felt better in my God-damned life!" His eyes had hardened and a half grin was on his face. He stared at Art as though using his eyes to penetrate his skull. Then he let his gaze sweep around the bar, looking to see what chance there might be for a little excitement.

Johnny picked up the drink in front of him, took a hard swallow, then spit it out onto the floor. "What sort of crap was the chickenshit drinking?" he said, oblivious to the looks of the other patrons.

"Hey, you!" shouted Johnny, motioning to the bartender. "Give me a God-damn double rum and Coke and get rid of this crap!"

Art was stunned by the sudden and complete change that had come over his boss. He had always known him to be a cool, even-tempered, conservative man who never raised his voice or became angry. The only explanation he could think of was that his boss might be leading a double life. Perhaps he carefully controlled himself in the office, but after work, when he decided to let go, he could be as wild and boisterous as any of them. He was shocked, yet he felt somewhat flattered that his boss would be willing to let down in front of him.

Art glanced at his watch as Johnny swallowed his drink. "It's almost time for your flight," he said. "You'd better get over to your gate. I'm going to drive back to the hotel. Have a nice flight."

"To hell with the airplane!" said Johnny. "Let's go out and ball it up tonight! I know a place in town that's loaded with swinging broads. And don't worry about money, Dana brought plenty with him."

Art had been thinking of hitting the hotel bar after he left the airport anyway, so the idea of drinking at someone else's expense seemed a pleasant one. He was also curious about what his boss was like when he relaxed after work. He knew that a relationship developed under those circumstances could be advantageous to his career.

The two of them drove to a hotel bar Johnny knew about. It was a swingers' hangout just beginning to fill for the evening. Johnny ordered drinks for himself and Art. He finished his, then ordered a second as well as drinks for two girls he had noticed at the end of the bar. When the bartender took the liquor to the girls, Johnny moved down to get acquainted.

Johnny, Art, and the two girls moved to a table. Art was a good dancer so he began dancing with the girls one at a time while Johnny sat drinking. After a time Johnny said, "Hey, girls, you know who you've been talking to?"

"No," said the girls.

"You're talking to the Devil himself! I've come here to recruit a couple of gals to be witches. You interested in having the power of a witch?"

"Sure," said the girls, laughing at him. "We'd like to have the power of a witch."

"Okay. The four of us have to go to a motel and I'll put you through the ritual indoctrination."

The girls laughed again. "Let's see how the evening goes," they said.

Johnny kept the joke going while they drank and danced for another hour. Then one of the girls said, "I don't know about going to a motel, but let's get out of here so we can talk about it."

"Fine," said Johnny, rising from the table. "We'll go grab a motel room and see if the girls qualify."

Art remained awed by Dana's actions. He had never seen him behave in such a manner. However, by then he had enough drinks in him to be game for anything. He couldn't imagine the girls falling for the phony line Johnny was handing them, but if they were interested in going to a motel, who was he to say no?

"Which way do we go now?" he asked, behind the wheel of the rented Thunderbird. "I don't know my way around this city."

"Hell!" said Johnny, sitting in back, his arms around one of the girls. "You don't have to know your way around. Just start driving and pull into the first damned motel you see."

"Maybe we should stop and have another drink first," said one of the girls, a little apprehensively.

"Let's have a drink afterwards!" said Johnny firmly. The girl studied him a moment, then agreed. "Okay, we're game for anything."

The car had gone only four blocks when the boisterous Johnny suddenly became quiet. His body relaxed, the tension drained from his muscles, his twisted smile disappeared from his face. He became calm, peaceful, the suggestion of violence disappearing entirely.

"Art, as soon as you can move over into the right-hand

lane, pull up to the curb and let the girls out," said Phil. His voice was steady, not so deep as Johnny's and totally unemotional. It was the voice of a self-confident man who felt himself in complete control of any situation. The radical change in him immediately electrified the car. The girls stared at him in disbelief.

"Don't argue with me or question what I'm about to say," said Phil, talking to the girl sitting next to him. "For your own sake and possible safety, I suggest that when Art pulls over, you leave the car and take a taxi back to the bar." He handed her a $5 bill to cover the expense.

"Drop the girls off at the corner?" said Art, stunned. "Why would I want to do a thing like that?"

"Art, please don't question my decision," said Phil. "Just do what I asked you to do." The tone of his voice carried such authority that Art felt he dare not argue. He knew he would have to settle for a cold shower that night.

Art pulled over to the curb. The girls were bewildered by Phil's behavior but realized he was serious. They got out of the car and started down the street. Phil also got out, then climbed into the front passenger seat.

"Take me straight to the airport," he said. "I want to see if I can get another flight out of here."

"My God," said Art, staring at him. "I've never seen anybody change his mind so fast."

"Don't argue with me, Art. Please do as I ask."

Art turned the car around and headed back to the airport. Before they had gone very far, he noticed his boss fidgeting on the seat. He was constantly shifting his position, looking out of first one side of the car and then the other. Periodically he would turn completely around, kneeling on the seat, his chin on the back rest, so he could look out the rear window. His eyes were wide and his face was flushed with excitement, much like the face of a child in an amusement park.

"Hi," said Peter when he realized Art was looking at him. His voice was high-pitched, almost squeaky. "Boy, isn't that Johnny bad?"

Art was shocked and a little annoyed by this bizarre behavior. "Who in the world is Johnny, Dana?" he asked.

"Oh, you know Johnny," said Peter. "He's the one who wanted to take those girls to the motel and do funny things with them." His body shuddered slightly as he tried to imagine what things Johnny might have done. "He's just not good at all."

Art was silent. He didn't know if his boss was drunk or crazy.

Peter looked around again, then asked, "Are you taking me to the airport?"

"That's where you told me to take you," said Art, coldly.

Peter became animated again, gesturing as he spoke. "Did you know that a long, long, long, long time ago I used to be able to fly without any airplane? I could fly anywhere I wanted to go."

Suddenly Peter looked embarrassed. "Oops," he said, bringing his hand to his mouth. "I guess I really shouldn't have told you that. You don't really know us, do you? I mean, you called me Dana and Dana isn't here. You probably don't even know what I'm talking about." He began giggling, cupping his hands over his face as though trying to hide.

Art was silent the rest of the way to the airport. He let Peter off, noticing once more how oddly he suddenly looked. "I'll see you the end of the week," he said.

Peter waved as Art started back to his hotel. "Pleasure meeting you!" he called.

Then Peter walked into the airport, his body bouncing with every step. Airports could be exciting places, especially if you had a pocket full of money. He knew that big airports always had amusement areas, and he decided he wanted to play one of the pinball machines.

Peter found the amusement area. He took a coin from his pocket, dropped it in a slot, and waited for the first ball to roll against the plunger. Then he fired it, watching it strike bells and buzzers, scoring points as it rolled its zig-zag course. His fingers tensed over the flipper levers. If he could keep the ball in the upper section he might score enough points to win a free bonus game!

The score began mounting: 10 points. 100 points. 200 . . . 500 . . . 1,000. . . .

"Crap!" said Johnny, moving briskly away from the machine. "That son-of-a-bitch Phil had to take over just when I was going to have some fun. And then that asshole kid . . . My God, what I need is to get this body all to myself. Those other bastards don't know how to live!"

He looked around him. "Back in the damned airport again," he said. He went to the bar, downed a quick drink, then started for the airport door. Perhaps those girls had returned to the singles hangout where he had first met them.

He moved quickly, his strides powerful, his body tensed with anger. His arms were taut and his hands were balled into fists. He felt like striking someone. If he couldn't find those girls again, he just might take the bar apart.

He put his hand up to open the outside door, then suddenly lowered it again. His face softened and his body relaxed. He turned and started back toward the ticket counter. His pace was slower, the sound of his shoes, moments before echoing as they struck the floor, now softened to a whisper. Phil was in control once more.

Phil asked about the next plane to his home town, then bought a one-way fare for the earliest departure time —nine the next morning. He went to the rest area, planning to spend the night in the airport to be certain Dana was able to return to his family.

It was after midnight when he sat down. Dana had been on the go all day and Johnny had been drinking heavily. Phil's tolerance to alcohol was quite low. He soon found himself drifting off to sleep. His head nodded against his chest, then jerked upright. His eyes narrowed and his face hardened. Johnny was back.

"Son-of-a-bitch can't handle liquor," Johnny laughed, studying the ticket Phil had purchased, then walking back to the ticket counter. "I want to change this to the next flight to Las Vegas."

"Certainly, Sir. There's a flight leaving in an hour."

For the next three days and two nights Johnny had his

usual gambling and sex spree. On the third night, when
Johnny finally fell asleep with a prostitute, Phil took over
once more. He climbed out of bed and put on his clothing,
being careful not to wake the prostitute.

"Hey, where you goin', honey?" asked the girl. She rolled
over so she could see him better, rubbing her eyes to wake
up.

"There's something I've got to get downstairs. I'll be
back in a minute. Don't go anywhere." Phil smiled at her,
then left the room with no intention of returning.

He had no intention of checking out before leaving the
motel. He didn't know what Johnny's bill might be and he
didn't care. The important thing was to get Dana back to
his family.

He inspected his wallet. It still contained $300 in cash.
He took a taxi to the airport and arranged for a flight
back home.

Dana awakened on the plane. His last memory was of
being in the Los Angeles airport. He assumed he had lost
just thirty or forty minutes, during which time he had obviously boarded the plane for home.

There was a magazine in the pouch in front of him and
Dana thumbed through it. He glanced at his watch again
and realized the flight was taking much longer than usual.
Normally the distance could be covered in an hour, but
they had already been flying twice that long. He wondered
if there was some sort of routing problem that had forced
them to fly a roundabout way.

When the plane finally landed at his home town airport,
he found his car and drove to the exit, handing the man
the ticket. The charge came to more than $7, several times
the daily rate. He paid it, trying not to show the shock he
felt. Once again he had lost several days. He hurried
home, trying to think of what he could say to Ann.

Dana still wasn't facing the truth about himself. He told
Ann that he had had to stay a few extra days. He said that
he had called her once but nobody had been home.

The sad part about Dana's lies was that they didn't

match his character. If he really had had to stay away that long, he wouldn't have let Ann worry. If there had been no answer when he had called, he would have called again and again until he had reached her or one of the kids. He cared for them too much to let them be concerned about his whereabouts.

Ann knew Dana was lying and it hurt her that he wouldn't confide in her. She didn't realize that he genuinely didn't know what happened during these periods.

"Steve Shaw called while you were gone," she told him. "He said he tried to reach you earlier in Los Angeles and was told you'd left three days ago." She watched Dana for his reaction. He tried to control his face so she wouldn't see the shame and guilt he felt for lying to her.

"Mr. Shaw was mistaken," he said quickly. "I only kept the first room I had for one night. Then I changed to a more comfortable one. Whoever Mr. Shaw talked to must not have noticed it."

Dana went to work the next day and immediately reported to Shaw's office. He explained that he had relatives in the Los Angeles area and had made a short vacation of the trip, visiting them after the opening session of the training program. He said he hadn't called because he had had nothing special scheduled for the week and hadn't thought it would matter very much anyway. He apologized for not being there when Shaw had tried to reach him.

Steve Shaw, an extremely conservative man, was upset by any deviation from normal policy. He felt that Dana should at least have called the office and left a number where he could have been reached. Yet he knew Dana had been responsible for the phenomenal growth of the corporation and was willing to admit that he deserved a rest.

When the other men who had gone to Los Angeles returned a few days later, Art went to Shaw's office to tell him about Dana's bizarre behavior. Dana was called into the office once more so Art could repeat the story to his face.

"Art's exaggerating," said Dana. "I was just kidding

around with him that night. I'm surprised he can't tell when somebody's joking around."

"That's not my idea of joking," said Art, angered by Dana's remarks. He thought his boss was crazy and he resented the way Shaw seemed to be supporting Dana. He decided he didn't want to continue working there under such circumstances. He quit on the spot.

Art's action upset Shaw even more. It was suddenly obvious to him that Dana was less skilled at handling interpersonal relations than he had thought. Still, one incident was not enough to base a major personnel change on. He would watch Dana more closely, that was all.

Oddly enough, when Dana did change jobs some time later, it was his own decision entirely. He had several advanced marketing ideas he wanted to implement. He felt that unless they were tried, the corporation would soon stop growing. But Steve Shaw was too conservative to listen seriously to them. If something hadn't been proven over and over again, he was not going to implement it.

Dana became disgusted. He knew he could do nothing more for the company if his ideas weren't tried. He felt he had to resign. His action was soon duplicated by a number of other staff members who agreed with his thinking. In addition, the insurance company that had been underwriting the corporation pulled out its financial support. They felt that Dana's skills were what had made the corporation what it was, and they weren't going to risk backing it without him. The move didn't break the firm—Dana's efforts had made it grow too big for that—but it did drastically reduce its size.

Dana sold his ten percent stock back to the company, taking a cash settlement. He had decided it was time to go into business for himself.

Through his contacts in the field, he was soon able to become a general agent for Mammoth Insurance Company. He received an exclusive northern California contract and opened his own office. He then hired a number of men and put them under his father, who had also left

Steve Shaw's firm. His father was given the title of District Manager—a move that was to prove quite costly.

His father decided that since Dana was footing the bills, he could be rather liberal with his use of the business facilities. He had a girl friend who had moved back to Washington, D.C., so he used the business telephone to call her daily. His phone bills alone ran several hundred dollars a month.

Dana wanted to make the business a success but he was seldom in the office. Most of the time Johnny would take over on the way to work. He spent his days chasing booze and broads instead of letting Dana chase clients. As a result there was no leadership for the agents and not enough capital to meet the expenses his father was running up.

After a few months everything Dana had hoped to build came crashing down. The business was facing bankruptcy. He was four months behind on his house payments and foreclosure proceedings had already been started. His home life was extremely tense.

Dana couldn't stand the abuse of Johnny and Peter any longer. He didn't know what was causing his periods of amnesia or what he was doing when he had them, but he knew he couldn't continue with them much longer. For the second time in his life he went to see a psychiatrist.

CHAPTER 17

Dana was nervous when he entered the office of Dr. William Heinrich. While he recognized that he needed help, he was frightened of what the doctor's diagnosis might be. He had visions of being committed to an asylum somewhere, or otherwise having his life turned upside down. Yet he knew that the way he was living was a nightmare and had to end.

The doctor's office was simply furnished, almost sterile in appearance. Instead of a couch there was a large easy chair meant to help the patients relax. Dana remained tense throughout the first meeting, but he was completely open about his mental history. He told of the blackouts and the strange behavior people had noticed during his amnesia spells. He described the sudden depression that always preceded the amnesia, as well as everything else about his life that made it seem so different from other people's.

During the next several sessions Dana was encouraged to talk about anything that came into his head. He told about his life and the times he had found himself in Las

Vegas hotel rooms without knowing how he had gotten there.

After a few weeks of this, and a series of tests conducted by a psychologist, Dana was told he was a manic-depressive. The condition is characterized by periods of great elation and extreme depression; however, the radical mood shifts, occurring for no apparent reason, are normally not accompanied by amnesia. The diagnosis was incorrect—but Dana was pleased that someone had at last placed a label on his condition. To him it meant that he might be treatable; he might be able to lead a normal life at last.

The psychiatrist prescribed a combination of amphetamines to make him feel better when he was depressed and tranquilizers to keep him at a normal emotional level when he was highly elated. Dana tried to explain to him that he had no warnings when the blackouts were about to occur. The feeling of depression lasted only a second or two, a period far too short for him to be able to take the pills in time. He said that he would be feeling fine and suddenly discover that two weeks had passed during which he had done things he simply couldn't remember.

The doctor replied that Dana was talking nonsense. He must have more warning than a second or two because all manic-depressives did. He also said the amnesia was caused by Dana's desire to forget, not by any other factors.

For several months Dana tried to follow the doctor's advice. If he felt the slightest bit sad he would immediately take an amphetamine; when he began to feel happy he would pop a tranquilizer to bring him down again. This restricted his emotional range even more than normal, but it didn't stop the blackouts. Johnny and Peter came and went at will. Dana's mental health had not changed.

The drug therapy had been going on for less than a year when an incident occurred one day that ended that phase of Dana's psychiatric treatment. He had come home from work, kissed Ann, and gone into the bedroom to change from his suit into more casual clothing. As he finished buttoning his shirt he felt the brief wave of depression. For a second he thought of the amphetamines, but before he could go for them Johnny was in control.

"So how's Dana's little angel?" said Johnny, walking into the kitchen and putting his arms around Ann. She recognized that he had changed from his appearance and the way he was talking; she moved from his grasp, wary.

"Listen, angel, I'm going to give you the thrill of your lifetime. I'm going to take you all the way to Lake Tahoe." He described in intimate detail the orgy of sex and gambling he planned, pacing back and forth in the kitchen as he talked, his hands waving excitedly. His deep voice seemed almost to be spitting out the perversions he intended to enjoy with Dana's wife.

Ann was past the point of being shocked by Johnny. For the children's sake, however, she had to do something to quiet him down.

"I can't wait," she said, forcing a smile. "But we don't want to have the children underfoot. Let me call a baby sitter so we can leave tonight."

Ann telephoned Dr. Heinrich, who promised to come right over. Then she returned to the kitchen while Johnny amused himself by describing the sex tricks he intended to try.

Dr. Heinrich arrived after what seemed to Ann an interminable length of time. She answered the doorbell with relief.

Johnny recognized the psychiatrist even though he, himself, had never visited his office. He was livid with rage. He had offered Ann the chance of a lifetime. He had been willing to overcome all the hard feelings he had had toward her after she had refused to have anything to do with him over the years. He had made an effort to give her the kind of thrill Dana could never provide. And after all that she had had the nerve to call the doctor! He grabbed her arm and started to strike her. The doctor managed to separate them.

Johnny stepped back and suddenly realized how ridiculous the situation was. He began laughing. "You bastards think I'm Dana, don't you? That chickenshit wouldn't have the guts to plan the trip I'm going to take." He turned to the doctor and said, "As for you, what the hell do you think you're doing? I'm Johnny, not Dana. Dana's the only one who's ever been a patient of yours."

Then he paused and studied the doctor's face a moment. Perhaps with a few drinks in him the doctor might not be such a bad guy. After all, he heard weird things from people every day. Since the bitch Dana married obviously wasn't going to go with him, maybe he and the doc could dig up a little action.

"Let's you and me go to a bar, Doc," said Johnny, taking the astounded psychiatrist by the arm. "I'm going to buy you a drink and tell you all about Dana and me."

Ann let out a sign of relief when the two of them left the house. Once again the children had avoided hearing Dana in one of his "moods." She had tried hard over the years to keep them unaware of what was happening to their father. Even when he was in jail she had tried to keep her concern from showing. She had always told the children Dana was away on a business trip. Dana was so kind and attentive towards them when he was "himself" that she hadn't wanted to say anything that might alienate the children from him. His tremendous kindness during those good periods was what had convinced her that he was worth trying to live with. It was only nights like tonight when she wondered if it would be better to leave him.

Johnny gave the psychiatrist the ride of his life. He put his foot to the floor and didn't let up on the gas until they reached a bowling alley thirty miles away. The car went through red lights and around oncoming traffic, took corners with the wheels squealing, and peeled rubber at every stop.

"Slow down, Dana. I'm in no hurry," said Dr. Heinrich. Reason with this crazy man, he thought to himself. Assume control. That's the professional way to handle this.

Johnny pulled into the parking lot of the bowling alley,

slamming on his brakes and stopping just before the car hit a post. "I thought we'd do a little bowling. They got beer here and sometimes you can pick up a few good-looking broads in these joints." He nudged the doctor in the ribs, then put his hand on the man's shoulder and guided him inside.

"I'm sorry, Sir, but this is league night. All the lanes are taken and I'm afraid they will be until closing time."

"We'll have to go somewhere else, Dana," said Dr. Heinrich, somewhat apprehensive about getting back in the car with Johnny at the wheel.

"Screw this!" said Johnny. "I came here to bowl and I'm God-damn well going to do it." He leaped the wall separating the spectators from the bowling teams, picked up a ball, and walked to the alley. A man was about to bowl but Johnny knocked him aside. Then he hurled his ball, sending it at high speed straight down the alley. It was a perfect strike.

"Top that, you sons-of-bitches!" he said, laughing at the astounded team members. He leaped back over the wall, took the doctor, and guided him to the car.

"Perhaps a little slower this time, all right?" said the doctor

"Hell, Doc," Johnny replied, guiding the car from the lot. "If these babies weren't meant to go fast they wouldn't have put such big numbers on the speedometer. You just hold onto your hat." He laughed as he roared the few blocks to the waterfront, stopping in front of a bar.

Waterfront bars are great places for fights, and Johnny started one the moment he got inside. The psychiatrist was shocked, especially since Johnny seemed to want him to get involved as well. He had had enough of this obvious lunatic. He sneaked out, called a cab, and left the area. Johnny stayed behind to drink until the bar closed at 2 A.M. There were no hard feelings among the men he had beaten. Brawling was just another part of having a good time for most of the patrons.

The following day Dana saw Dr. Heinrich, who told him

what had happened the night before. The doctor was irate. He had never been so embarrassed and humiliated in his life. He informed Dana that the only way he would consider keeping him as a patient would be if Dana would submit to a lobotomy.

Dana was shocked. A lobotomy involves the cutting away of a portion of the brain, sometimes leaving the patient nothing more than an even-tempered vegetable. It is considered the most extreme measure that can be taken in a mental case. It was certainly not an operation to which Dana would submit. He felt that whatever was wrong with him, somewhere, sometime, he would learn what it was and what could be done to cure it.

That ended his sessions with Dr. Heinrich. Ten more years would pass before he would seek psychiatric help again.

CHAPTER 18

Dana soon realized that his insurance career in California was over. Johnny had given him a reputation in the business of being an unpredictable hothead, and no company would hire him, even though they all knew that he was highly skilled and often seemed highly motivated.

The furniture business, too, seemed to offer little hope. Dana was qualified to run an appliance or furniture store, but the only jobs available were low-paying sales positions for which he was over-qualified. Most of them were dead-end situations, so that even if he were to become a company's top salesman he still could earn only a small fraction of the income he had once known. The store owners were reluctant to hire him, fearing he would quickly become dissatisfied.

It seemed time to move on. Dana and Ann stayed up all night discussing their situation and the possibilities for their future. They agreed it was time to go to a new state, where they could get a fresh start. They would sell all their nonessential belongings and use the money to relocate in a new city.

The first question was where to go. All their relatives were in or near that part of California where they were then living. They wanted to remain close enough to be able to return quickly should an emergency arise. They decided that 1,000 miles was the maximum they would travel.

Dana was also without a driver's license; it had been suspended once again because of Johnny's drunk driving. All the border states had agreed not to issue a license to anyone whose previous license had been revoked by California. Therefore they would have to move at least two states away.

Dana and Ann took a map and drew a half circle indicating the agreed-on 1,000-mile radius. Within the half circle were Phoenix and numerous other cities of various sizes. But the one that had the greatest appeal was Salt Lake City. They had been through the area in the past and liked the climate as well as the mountainous beauty of the Rockies.

Ann made arrangements to take the children and move into her sister's extremely large home. Dana would go alone to Salt Lake City to find a job and a place to stay.

It took a week for Dana to find a job. He answered every advertisement he could find, then grabbed the first position that was offered to him. It was a clerk's job in a 7-11 store, and it required that he put in 48 hours a week. He also found a house for $125 a month and immediately called Ann, telling her to come.

The next nine months went fairly smoothly. Dana was able to get a Utah driver's license and somehow save enough money from his salary to buy a used car.

His skills soon became obvious to his employer. He was promoted to assistant store manager, then store manager, then assistant district manager for twelve stores. Each promotion brought a fairly large increase in salary. His family was able to live modestly but comfortably, and he began paying off their bills. Moreover, the children, especially, loved Utah. The climate was different from what they had known and they enjoyed the mountains.

But the serenity of his Utah career would not last long. A district manager position became available and the heads of the company called together all the assistant managers of the mountain states for a meeting in Salt Lake City. There were twelve in all, including Dana. During the meeting three finalists were selected for the position. Dana was one of the three.

The meeting lasted until 12:30 A.M. Dana was tired but happy as he began the drive home. He had gone about a mile when he lost consciousness and Johnny took over.

Johnny had been unusually quiet during the past few months, but he was determined to change all that now. It was time for him to bust loose and have a ball. He drove to the nearest 7-11 store and went directly to the safe. Dana had a key for it in his pocket. Johnny found the key, opened the safe, and emptied it of $1,200 in currency.

"Might as well do things up right," thought Johnny after stuffing the money in his pockets. "I'll make those bastards hate that chickenshit Dana." He began pulling boxes of food from the shelves and hurling cupcakes and doughnuts to the floor. He grabbed a bottle of soda pop, shook it violently, then threw it against the wall. It exploded, the pressure from the carbonation sending the sticky liquid flying throughout the store. He knocked over display racks and tossed magazines into the air. Then he got back into the car and drove to the Nevada border, where he began drinking and gambling in a town just over the state line.

Johnny knew of a whorehouse in the area and decided to visit it that morning. But even Johnny discovered that night that there were limits to his enormous energy. He had gone twenty-four hours without sleep, and found himself unable to perform with the girls. Instead he bought them all drinks and they sat talking together the rest of the morning.

Johnny didn't get to sleep until that evening. Then he took a motel room and collapsed on the bed.

It was early the following morning when he was awakened by a loud knock on the door. "Open up! It's the police!"

"Damn it all," said Johnny, submerging and letting Dana take control.

"Open up in there!"

Dana looked around the room, totally confused. It was obvious he was in a motel room and just as obvious that someone was trying to get inside.

"This is the police! If you don't open the door we'll use the pass key. There are men all around the building. There's no way to escape."

Escape? thought Dana. From what? He hadn't done anything wrong. He rose from the bed and started for the door.

"I'm coming," he called. "You woke me up. I'll be right there."

"Dana Hawksworth?" said the detective when he entered the room.

"Yes."

"We have a warrant for your arrest."

"Arrest?" said Dana. "What did I do?" His heart was beating rapidly. He knew he had had a blackout but this was the first time he had done anything serious enough to warrant the police coming for him. He wondered if he had hurt someone.

"You're being charged with grand theft."

Gradually Dana was able to learn what had happened; the knowledge sickened him. He had never abused a trust before.

He had been appreciative of the chance the store chain had given him. He wouldn't consciously do anything to betray their faith in him. Yet apparently he had.

Dana was taken to jail and held for a week until extradition to Utah could be arranged. Then he was picked up by the Utah Highway Patrol and taken back to Salt Lake City. There he was arraigned, charged with grand theft, and held under $5,000 bail. Fortunately Ann was able to raise the $550 fee needed to pay a bondsman and he was released.

"This is it, Dana," said Ann, tears in her eyes. "This is the final straw. I love you and I believed in you with all my heart. But just when things seem to be finally working themselves out, you go and do something stupid. I've been humiliated too often to continue. I'm taking the children and going to live with my parents in California. The children don't know what a mess you're in and I'm going to try to keep them from finding out. You've been a loving father. I'll say that for you. But it's just not enough any more."

Ann packed her belongings and left the state. Dana felt helpless. He had committed a crime he knew nothing about. He had lost his wife, possibly for good. He was a failure at everything he did, though he didn't understand why. He became extremely depressed and Phil took control.

Phil had no time to waste on self-pity. He appeared before the court and asked permission to be his own attorney. Then he went to see the District Attorney. Court trials were expensive and Dana's crime was not one to make headlines. His record with the food stores had been so good that they were not anxious to prosecute, even though they did want him to undergo some punishment for what he had done. As a result, Phil was able to plea bargain, getting the charge reduced to one of simple theft—a misdemeanor. Bail was lowered to $500 and Phil pleaded guilty.

He was not sentenced immediately. An appointment, one week later, was set with the probation department. Final sentencing would take place in two weeks, giving the probation officer time to file a report on what he felt Dana's punishment should be.

When the report was made, it recommended that Dana be given ninety days in jail. If the system had proceeded normally, he would shortly have begun serving his time.

"Son-of-a-bitch!" said Johnny, wrestling control away from Phil. "That bastard wants to put us in jail. I've had enough of his crap! I'm getting out of here."

Johnny got into Dana's car and headed for Nevada once more. He was stopped by the Highway Patrol for doing 95 along the way, but the officers who stopped him never realized he was a fugitive from justice and let him get away. After he reached Nevada he spent three days gambling and drinking. He also picked up a girl at a local bar and took her back to the hotel with him.

The girl was extremely attractive. She said as she undressed and climbed into bed that she was part Indian. Johnny was just removing his pants when Phil suddenly took over.

The transformation shocked the girl. She saw the body and voice change. The wild man she had accompanied to the room was gone. Instead, Phil told her that he had suddenly remembered something important and would have to leave at once. He dressed and walked from the room, leaving the speechless girl staring wide-eyed after him.

Phil returned to Salt Lake City, taking a room in a cheap hotel. He used the hotel's stationery to write a note to Dana. It read: "Leave for California the first thing in the morning. Join your wife in California. They will not extradite you for a misdemeanor. Stay out of Utah for seven years. Signed: Your Friend." Then he climbed into bed and went to sleep. In the morning it was Dana who awakened.

Dana read the letter, not knowing who had written it. He did not question the message, though. He got into his car and drove back to California.

Ann was reluctant to reconcile with him when he first appeared. She and the children were living with her parents in a cabin in the mountains of northern California. The life wasn't pleasant, but at least it was no longer filled with the anxiety of never knowing what Dana would be like from one minute to the next.

The children, however, were very happy to see their father—a fact that had great influence on Ann. After discussing it with Dana at great length she agreed finally to try once more. She wasn't certain it was the right move to make, but she loved him too much not to give him one more chance.

Dana found a job as a sewing machine repairman, using his Utah license in order to drive. He didn't tell his employer that he could not get a California license. He explained that he was planning to get one and just hadn't had the chance. The pay was fairly low but Ann was able to find work as a maid in a nearby motel. Together they hoped once again to get ahead of the ever-mounting bills caused by Johnny's misadventures.

Johnny was fairly quiet during this period, but Peter was making frequent appearances at night. He was becoming increasingly serious about his poetry and spent many hours trying to improve it.

For more than thirty years Dana had been finding this poetry and by now he had grown to accept it. He assumed that it must have been written by his subconscious mind, perhaps while he was half asleep—although he didn't know why the handwriting was so different from the way his usually looked. He just took its existence as being something natural; if he had ever suspected otherwise, the implication would have been that there was something seriously wrong with his mind, and he didn't want to face that possibility.

Dana had some free time in the evenings. When he read in the paper that there would be an adult education course in creative writing at a local school, he decided to sign up for it and take Peter's work with him. Every time the class was given an assignment, Dana would turn in whichever of Peter's writings seemed appropriate.

By the time the third class rolled around, Peter was very much aware of what Dana was doing. He decided that the education was being wasted on Dana and soon got in the habit of taking over the body on the way to the class. He would enter the school, bouncing happily along as he moved through the corridors, his eyes bright and his face eager with anticipation. He would listen carefully to everything the teacher said, then practice writing all night after the class. Dana was losing a lot of sleep as a result, though he never realized what caused his morning tiredness.

Johnny liked the idea of the classes as well. At first he

just observed what was happening. Dana would start to go
to the class, black out, then find himself driving home with
a notebook filled with notes in someone else's handwriting.
He assumed he had attended, though he had no memory of
it.

But then Johnny realized that he could take control directly from Peter. Peter was terrified of Johnny, but so
excited about the class that he was able to retain control
until it was over. After that, though, instead of Dana re-
gaining control, Johnny would take over and spend a few
hours bar-hopping. Three times during the nine months
Dana was enrolled in the course he awakened in motels
with girls beside him. Each time he got dressed and left,
quite upset. He was not the type to cheat on his wife.

While Dana was working for the sewing machine company he received a call one day from an employment
agency with which he had registered. They had a job for
him stocking shelves in a supermarket in a small resort
town just a few miles from where he was living. The pay
was similar but the job offered an opportunity for advancement that he did not have where he was currently
employed. He decided to accept it.

At the same time Ann found a new job working with an
electronics firm. Her pay increased and she eventually
more than doubled her income, becoming a quality-control
inspector.

Dana was determined to become successful with the supermarket. He became quite popular with the customers
and displayed a willingness to work, and in just three
years advanced to the position of store manager.

During the time Dana worked at the grocery store,
Johnny did not come out often enough to get him in much
trouble. Usually he would take off for a brief orgy of gambling in Nevada. He kept Dana in debt but avoided getting arrested or otherwise causing serious trouble.

Dana became increasingly involved in community affairs while working at the grocery store. He became a Boy
Scout Troop leader as well as heading the 4-H Clubs in the

area. He organized a parents' club in the high school to act as a lobbying body with the Board of Education to try to improve the quality of the teaching.

The community affairs brought Dana closer to his family as well. His daughter was active in 4-H and his older son was in the Scout troop. They took pride in their father's interest in what they did. Ann began to feel that her decision to stay with Dana had been the right one to make.

But Dana was concerned about this new reputation he was suddenly acquiring with his children. Ann had done such a good job of protecting them from knowledge of their father's "moods" that he felt they might get a distorted picture of him. He feared that if they thought of him as being all good, they would one day learn that he was not and become disillusioned and bitter.

To prevent that from happening, he told them he had a drinking problem that had plagued him for many years. He explained that when he drank too much he was like a different person. He said it had caused him serious problems over the years and he was trying very hard to overcome it. He stressed that it was not something he had been able to lick. With this preparation, he felt, they would be less likely to be hurt if they ever did encounter the type of person he had been told he was during his blackouts.

Johnny, as usual, resented Dana's success. For some reason he totally ignored the involvement in community affairs, even though they resulted in Dana's name being in the area newspapers and his making appearances on radio and television. What he wanted was to get him fired from his job again, for getting Dana fired hurt both him and Ann, a woman Johnny hated for not yielding to him.

It was eight A.M. and Dana was driving the two miles to the grocery store. He felt a sudden depression, slumped slightly, and sent the car momentarily out of its lane. In seconds Johnny was in control. He pulled to the right, checked the flow of traffic, and made a U-turn. He drove the fifteen miles to a nearby community where he went to the bank and emptied Dana's checking account of $150.

Johnny knew some drinking spots in San Jose, several miles away. He drove there, drinking and fighting in several bars. Finally he picked up a woman and took her to a motel for the night.

Johnny was not certain just how much control he had at the moment, so he decided not to risk going to sleep. Instead he stayed awake with the woman all that night, then dumped her in an early-morning bar. He had a few more drinks, then cashed several bad checks at a number of different businesses.

After exploring the remaining bars around town, he decided to do a little traveling. He began speeding toward the outskirts of the city but was stopped for drunken driving before he could make it out of town. He was taken to jail until he could hire a bondsman to bail him out. He stayed in control the entire time, despite his hatred for drunk tanks. He knew he would soon be released and wanted to be able to continue his fun.

Bail was just $50 and Johnny was held only four hours. As soon as he was released he got into Dana's car and hit a few more bars. Then he drove to Los Angeles hoping to find more action. He arrived at 6 A.M.

It had been forty-eight hours since he had last slept, and he was tired. He had always had a high flow of adrenalin that kept him active, but this time it was not enough to overcome the tremendous exhaustion affecting his body. He was forced to take a motel room, collapsing on the bed for essential sleep.

Johnny was relieved to awaken at four that afternoon. He had been worried that Phil might take control while he was unconscious. He went down to the strip in Los Angeles, drinking in a number of bars.

He was in a traveling mood. He went from Los Angeles to San Diego, drinking in the bars near the naval base for two days, then headed south once more, stopping finally in Tijuana, Mexico.

But the Mexican trip was one too many for Johnny. The strain of the past several days had weakened him enough for Peter to take control. Peter found himself in a motel room in a country he had never visited. It was a fact that delighted him.

Peter left the car at the motel and began walking the streets. He was a poor driver even when he knew the roads. He wasn't going to take the chance of driving in another country.

All the sights and sounds of Mexico were strange and wondrous to Peter. He cocked his head to listen to the cadence of the Spanish language, delighting in the strange, melodic sounds. He ran his hands over the pots and other craft goods available in the various shops. And everywhere he walked the people seemed friendly, smiling at him as he passed. The fact that his wide-eyed look and bouncy walk made him seem rather simple-minded went unnoticed by him.

The heat of the day began to feel a little severe so Peter went into one of the nicer restaurants to have a beer. There was a young American couple in the restaurant and he struck up a conversation with them. The man was black and the woman was white. They had been touring the country together.

Peter was fascinated by the twosome. He had never known an interracial couple before and was anxious to learn of their experiences. He wanted to know what they thought of each other and how people reacted to them. He explained that he was a poet and that their love, transcending society's hate, would make a beautiful poem.

The couple seemed to enjoy Peter. They appreciated his open questioning, totally devoid of any prejudice. He seemed strange, more childlike than adult, but they spent considerable time in his company.

Peter never did write the poem he had in mind, however. By late afternoon Johnny was strong enough to take control of the body once again.

Johnny immediately headed for the bars Peter had avoided. He kept his activities to a minimum, though, knowing that Mexican police had a different system from the one used by police in the States. If he got thrown into a Mexican jail for fighting, neither he nor Dana nor even Phil would be able to get him out.

By late afternoon he had had his fill of Mexico. He re: turned to San Diego, hitting the few night spots he had missed on the way south.

Soon he grew bored with what was available in California. He got back into the car and started driving to Las Vegas. A little gambling seemed to be the ideal way to spend the next twenty-four hours.

He was in a hurry to reach Nevada. He accelerated quickly, then kept the pedal to the floor. He was doing 100 when he saw the Highway Patrolman coming up behind him, his lights flashing and sirens blaring.

For a moment he thought about trying to outrun the Patrolman. He kept his foot on the gas, considering what might happen. The pigs would probably throw up a road block somewhere. And the chickenshit never bought himself cars with enough power to outrun the guy behind him. There was really no choice. He took his foot off the gas and gently braked the car to a stop by the side of the highway.

Johnny was arrested for drunken driving. He raised hell with the officers but did not resist when they put him in the San Diego Jail. He stayed in control when he fell asleep, then let Dana awaken the following morning.

Dana had no idea where he was, though he recognized the fact that he was in a drunk tank. He had awakened too many times in too many different jails not to know that.

Most of his possessions had been taken by the police for safekeeping. However, when he felt in his pocket he found a copy of the form detailing the charge against him as well as the list of personal items the police were holding. Both were dated, so he was able to orient himself.

Dana phoned Ann to tell her where he was. He saw from the property slip that he still had enough cash to get out of jail. The bond fee came to $55. Dana paid the money, then got in his car and headed north. He had $30 left in his pocket, enough to cover gas and food for the next twelve hours.

It was also enough for Johnny to get to Las Vegas, a fact he realized before Dana could get as far as Los Angeles. Johnny took control and turned the car toward Nevada once more.

His route took him across miles of California desert. The monotony of the endless sand began to affect him. He became tired, fighting to stay awake. He felt himself slipping . . . slipping. . . .

"My God, where am I now?" wondered Dana, looking around. He eased his foot off the accelerator, bringing the speed down to the legal limit. There was sand all around him; it was difficult to orient himself. He didn't know where he was or how much time had passed.

After a few minutes he realized that he was on his way out of state. He turned the car around and started back for Los Angeles. Two miles down the road he saw a roadside stand where he bought a cup of coffee and learned the date. He was relieved that his amnesia had lasted only a couple of hours this time.

Dana returned to his car and started down the road. But even with the coffee, that endless sand began making him sleepy too. He felt depressed and, a moment later, Johnny was back in charge.

Johnny made another U-turn and drove all the way to Las Vegas, where he managed to cash $50 checks at a half dozen different places. Then he headed for the tables, trying his luck at everything from crap to the one-armed bandits.

Luck was with Johnny that night. Everything he tried seemed to put him a little more money ahead. He spent three days in the best hotels, eating the most expensive food, and still had $1,100 in his wallet—$800 more than when he had started.

Johnny began drinking a few rounds in celebration of his good fortune. A woman walked up to him and said, "Mind if someone celebrates with you?"

The woman had just been granted a divorce. She was in Las Vegas to wait for her papers and to have a little fun.

Johnny was delighted to drive the woman back to California, stopping at her trailer home in a small desert community.

Peter stretched and yawned when he awakened. As he moved, his body bumped against a naked woman sleeping soundly beside him. He jumped back, rolling off the mattress and onto the floor. His eyes were wide and his face was flushed. He had never been in bed with a woman before.

Hesitantly he raised the sheet to get a better look at her. "She's naked," he thought, quickly dropping the sheet and turning his head away. "Oh, my goodness. She must be one of those naughty ladies Johnny does funny things with." He glanced over at her again, then diverted his eyes.

"I can't stay here," Peter thought. "She might wake up and think I should do funny things with her too. She might. . . . " His face went beet red.

Peter found his clothing and dressed hastily. "Maybe if I'm real quiet and sneak out of here she won't wake up."

He tiptoed to the door, then slipped quietly from the trailer. He saw Dana's car and reluctantly got inside. "If I didn't have to spend so much time in this body, I could fly home like I used to do," he thought, starting the car. It sputtered, died, and had to be started again. The engine was beginning to flood. It took a moment to turn over. Peter found himself holding his breath until it roared into life. He released the brake and drove jerkily onto the road.

Peter reached another small community several miles down the road. There he discovered an all-night restaurant where he ordered a cup of coffee and sat down to collect his thoughts.

There was no one else in the restaurant, so he began talking with the cook. He asked the man how he came to be there and was fascinated by the cook's enthusiasm for the area. It seemed so desolate and isolated that Peter was surprised to learn how deeply the residents could love it.

Peter decided to remain in the desert area, driving from one small community to another, talking with the people about their lives. He told them that he was a writer who was gathering information about desert living. The people thought him a harmless character and were quite friendly with him, answering all his questions and occasionally buying him coffee or a sandwich.

After several days in the desert Peter misjudged the driving conditions and rolled off the road, getting the car stuck in the sand. He tried every way he knew to get it out but nothing worked. He sat down and a few moments later Phil was back in charge.

Phil had no trouble getting the car out of the sand and, back on the highway, headed toward home. He wanted to submerge and let Dana take control but recognized that Dana was too weak to fight Johnny and Peter. He felt it was his duty to get everyone safely back to Dana's house. He was certain Ann would be worried about Dana and did not want him delayed any further. There was no time to waste. Phil drove straight through until he reached home.

Phil told Ann he was sorry about what had happened. He explained that he was working to solve the problem, though not telling her that he and Dana were two different personalities.

Ann couldn't accept Phil's explanation. It was just another case of getting her hopes raised by Dana's success only to have him ruin everything by taking off for Nevada. She said that she no longer was able to cover for him with his boss; moreover the children were now of an age to realize things weren't right.

Phil said he was going to explain the unusual problem to the children. He stressed that he was going to work things out.

Ann was bothered by the way Phil was talking. He seemed genuinely concerned about what had happened and about her feelings in the matter. Yet he also seemed somewhat cold. It was as though he were a casual observer instead of the person with whom there was a problem. She still thought she was talking with Dana.

Phil gathered the children together in the living room.

He pretended to be Dana and told them once more that he had a periodic drinking problem linked with memory lapses. He explained that there were times when he wasn't even aware he had a problem; that night, however, his memory was working well. He was aware there were serious difficulties and he was doing everything in his power to resolve them.

The children seemed pleased to be treated as equals in being told about their father's difficulty. They respected him for telling them and genuinely believed in his ability to solve his problem. Only Ann was unconvinced. She had simply been through this too many times before.

CHAPTER **19**

The next several months were hectic ones for Dana. He lost his job with the grocery store just as Johnny had planned, then ran through a series of other jobs in the areas of admissions counseling and financial services for business schools. Finally he began to rise in the latter field, periodically switching schools to advance himself. But this, too, came to an end one day after he had risen to a top position with the northern California branch of a chain of business schools. The chain was going to become a franchise operation and one of the corporate executives had flown to California from the Seattle home office just to see Dana. He wanted to offer Dana his choice of either a franchise or the position of executive vice-president in charge of training for all the schools.

Dana's success was too much for Johnny to take. He gained control of the body as Dana drove to the meeting.

Johnny delighted in ridiculing the corporate executive who had come to see Dana. He insulted him, cursed and carried on like a wild man. Before the day was over, Dana was out of a job.

Once more success had been taken from his grasp. There was no longer any way he could excuse what had been happening to him. He had to admit there was no rational explanation for his memory lapses and erratic behavior. Something was wrong with his mind. He decided to see his family doctor for a referral to a psychiatrist.

Dana's family physician knew that he had just lost his job. He suggested a tax-supported mental health program run by the county hospital. The program consisted of group therapy treatment involving psychiatrists, psychologists, and social workers.

The county program had its good as well as bad points. Some of the staff members were highly skilled professionals who did a great deal of good for the patients in their care. Others were sadly lacking in ability. They seemed to have entered the field to try to better understand their own problems. It was Dana's misfortune to be treated by a doctor who proved less than competent.

After a few days of individual and group meetings, the doctor decided that what was wrong with Dana was that he hated his father.

"Dana Hawksworth, will you please come up in front of the group?" asked the doctor, smiling. He set a chair in front of Dana and placed a pillow on the seat. Then he handed Dana a tennis racquet and said, "The pillow on this chair is your father. I want you to imagine that he is there in front of you. Can you picture him where the pillow is?"

Dana said he could see him.

"Good. Now I want you to hit the pillow as hard as you can, over and over again. And in your mind I want you to think that you're really hitting your father, whom you hate." The doctor continued smiling.

This was ridiculous, thought Dana. He didn't hate his father. He didn't hate anyone. But he wasn't going to argue with the professional.

"All right. Beat the pillow. Hit it as hard as you can until you rid your body of all the hatred you feel toward your father. Only then will you be cured."

Dana half-heartedly hit the pillow. He wondered who was crazier—the patients or the psychiatrist.

The psychiatrist followed each unenthusiastic swing of the tennis racquet as it arced toward the pillow. His face was flushed with excitement; his body tense. He looked to Dana like some ancient Roman spectator viewing the battle of gladiators in an arena.

"Harder! Hit the pillow harder!" shouted the psychiatrist. "Beat it! Kill it!"

Dana used more force but it wasn't enough to satisfy the doctor. It also did nothing for his emotions. If anything he loved his father and was saddened that the two of them had never been able to develop a meaningful father-son relationship.

Dana realized that the doctor was going to keep him hitting the stupid pillow until he dropped from exhaustion. He decided to end the nonsense. He knew that the weakest part of the racquet was the narrow neck of the handle. He felt if he could strike that small section against the edge of the chair while he was thrashing at the pillow, perhaps he could break the racquet. The idea worked. The racquet split in two.

"You broke my tennis racquet!" said the psychiatrist, standing up, his face horrified, his body quivering with rage. "You were supposed to kill your father, not my racquet. Now you're going to have to buy me a new one."

Dana stared at the man for a minute, then returned to his place in the group. He decided that the patients had a definite edge over the staff in terms of sanity. It was time to quit the program. If help was available for his condition, it was not going to be found there.

The one good point that resulted from the hospital stay was that Dana again was diagnosed a manic-depressive. He and Ann began reading everything they could find on the condition, searching for a possible cure.

During this period his father became seriously ill for the first time in his life. He was sixty-four years old and married again, this time to a woman fifteen or twenty years younger than himself.

Dana's father had always believed in experiencing life in high gear. He had to be a big spender, the constant party goer, the wheeler-dealer. He would rather have a short, active life than an existence that required him to live without pressure. When he became ill, he worried that the future might have to be very different from his past.

He underwent a battery of tests to find out just what was wrong with him. He had emphysema, an enlarged heart, and numerous other problems. His body had simply been pushed too hard for too long, and it was falling apart on him. The doctor told him that the only way he could live was to spend a major part of each day relaxing. He would have to stop working, or at least slow his pace and take frequent vacations. It amounted to exactly that life style he had always sworn he would die before accepting.

That Friday after receiving news of his physical condition, he spent the day putting his affairs in order. He talked with his two sisters for the first time in many years. He saw his daughter, by then out of high school and living with a boy, and told her that if the two married, they would have his blessing. That night he went to sleep. He never awakened.

Earlier in the week, when Dana had visited him, he had revealed that he had a secret supply of sleeping pills. He had been given several prescriptions for the pills over a number of months and had taken one or two from each bottle and put them in a container only he knew about. He had said he would use them if he ever became an invalid; he didn't want to have people caring for him.

That Saturday morning Dana received a frantic call from his father's latest wife. She had found him dead in bed and didn't know what to do.

The words had barely been spoken when Phil took control as he had done when Dana's mother had died. He told Diane, his father's widow, that he would be right there. Then he drove to the home.

He went into the bedroom and examined his father's body, making certain the man was dead. He calmed Diane, then looked in the headboard for the bottle of sleeping pills. It was missing, though he discovered an empty container in the bathroom trash can. Apparently Diane had thrown them away so no one would suspect that it was a suicide.

Phil called the doctor and an ambulance came for the body. No autopsy was performed as his father had been a sick man. Phil arranged for the mortuary and the funeral.

That same Saturday Phil checked the strongbox his father kept at home. His father had once told Dana that the box contained his last will and testament and that he should look for it there when the time came. The strongbox had been forced open and the will was missing. Apparently Diane had wanted to be certain she would get her "rightful" share of the estate. She had been scheduled to get one of three insurance policies on his life but that obviously hadn't been enough; she had also wanted as many other tangible assets as possible. She would get them as part of her widow's share of the estate but would not have been eligible for them under the terms of the will. However, nothing could be proven and neither Dana nor his half-sister wanted to fight for any of the belongings. Phil insisted that certain things should go to his half-sister and he let Diane have everything else.

Dana's inheritance was perhaps the last put-down his father ever gave him, and it was strictly unintentional. There were three $10,000 life insurance policies—one for Diane, one for Dana's half-sister, and one for Dana. The first two had been purchased by Dana's father and the payments made in the usual way. But Dana's policy had been awarded as a bonus for his father's work with the insurance company. So long as his sales volume had remained high, the company had met the payments for him. But his illness had kept him from working to capacity long enough that the company had finally stopped payment on it. By the time he had died, the policy was no longer in force. The promised $10,000 was never paid.

Dana was not hurt by the loss of the insurance. He had

come to understand his father over the years. He didn't hate the man but there was no affection for him, either. He was content not to receive any money.

Dana attended the funeral because Phil thought he could handle that emotional experience. Dana, however, felt more like an observer than a participant. He felt as if he were sitting in a movie theater, watching the film of an event that was important to him, yet that didn't really involve him. The experience blunted the emotional strain that might otherwise have overwhelmed him.

Life seemed to go downhill after the funeral. Johnny went on one of his sprees and got Dana charged with drunk driving, resisting arrest and other crimes. Money was scarce and Dana's relationship with Ann grew quite strained. They both felt frustrated by their inability to handle Dana's "moods."

Dana's next job resulted from his answering an advertisement for an assistant manager of a store in a furniture chain More than a hundred people applied for the job, but Dana seemed the most versatile in terms of management experience. He was hired and six weeks later became Manager of the main store when the man who had held that position unexpectedly retired.

Once again his fortunes seemed to be on the rise. He continued to impress the furniture chain's owners during the next four months. His innovative procedures, ability to get along with fellow employees, and success in increasing sales resulted in yet another promotion. He was made General Manager of the entire chain. Once again he had reached a level of great respect and high income in his chosen field.

But Johnny, once more, had been watching his advancement with increasing disgust. He hated Dana and resented the idea that anybody would respect him so much. He decided it was time for him to do something to cut Dana back down to size.

He took over one evening about 5:30 P.M. when Dana was taking a dinner break in a small restaurant near the furniture store. He immediately slammed the remains of the sandwich Dana had been holding onto the plate and walked out of the building. The cashier called after him to pay for the food but he ignored her. That chickenshit Dana had ordered the sandwich, he hadn't. He had no intention of paying for it.

Johnny entered a bar, pushing one of the customers aside as he walked through the door. He ordered a drink, swallowed it as soon as it was served, then asked for a second.

"You drink those pretty fast," said the bartender. He smiled at Johnny.

"It's none of your God-damned business how fast I drink them. You just keep bringing them to me everytime I ask, you understand?" His voice was cold. The bartender felt Johnny's eyes were somehow penetrating his head.

"Yes, Sir," he said nervously.

Johnny ordered three more drinks, swallowing each one as fast as it was served. Then he left the bar and walked to the furniture store.

There was a lamp on display near the entrance to the store. Johnny knocked it to the floor as he stepped inside, causing a young couple looking at dinette sets to stare at him. "Hey, you sons-of-bitches, I'm here!" he said.

Frank Carter, son of the Executive Vice-President, left his office to see what was happening. He was shocked by the look on Johnny's face. He had been working with Dana for months and had never seen such an expression there before.

Johnny up-ended a couch and toppled a large armchair. "This place is like a morgue. You bastards ought to be happy I'm putting a little excitement into your lives," he said, laughing.

"Dana, are you crazy?" asked Frank. "What are you doing?"

"I'm busting up the joint, you snot-nosed bugger. What's it to you?"

"This isn't like you, Dana. Have you been drinking?"

Frank had long admired Dana's expertise in the business, and the two had become close friends despite a wide gap in their ages. He couldn't understand what was happening.

"The hell it's not like me. What do you think I am? I'm not like that little chickenshit who is such a damned goody-goody." There was a vase of dried flowers on one of the tables, part of a special display. Johnny knocked it to the floor.

"Dana, get hold of yourself. You're tearing up the place," said Frank, grabbing his arm. "Come into the office with me. We'll talk about whatever's bothering you."

"Get your God-damned hand off my arm," said Johnny coldly. He used his free hand to knock Frank back against a couch. The youth lost his balance and fell to the floor. He couldn't comprehend what had come over Dana. The man he thought was his friend was acting like a lunatic.

Johnny knocked over another chair, then said, "I don't know why an asshole like you is allowed to hang around this place. You've been sponging off your father for years. You couldn't make it on your own. You haven't got the guts or the brains. You're a nothing! A zero! Your kind makes me want to puke!"

When he had finished this tirade, Johnny marched out the door and headed for the nearest bar. He spent the rest of the night drinking while Frank and the other salespeople tried to clean up the mess he had made.

Dana was nauseated when he awakened. His head ached and his mouth felt as though he had been eating white paste. He turned to look at the clock on the headboard. It took a moment for his bloodshot eyes to focus and when they did he could barely read the numbers. It was 8:45.

"I'll never make it to work this morning," he thought numbly. He wondered about the previous night, trying to remember what he had done to make himself so sick. He couldn't remember a thing.

He struggled to his feet, leaning against the wall for support until the dizziness subsided. Then he realized that he still had his clothes on; the fact pleased him. Getting dressed was beyond his abilities for the moment.

Slowly he made his way to the kitchen. The house was empty. His daughter was in college and his two sons were in school. Ann would be at work.

The light in the refrigerator blinded him for a moment. He shielded his eyes from it and found a half gallon of milk. He took several swallows from the carton, then found a glass and filled it. His hand was shaking and he had to set the glass on the table to steady it.

The milk made Dana feel a little better. He was able to move to the wall phone, lift the receiver, and dial his employer.

"Lowery's Fine Furniture. May I help you?"

"Helen? This is Dana. I woke up with a case of the flu this morning. My stomach's upset and my head's spinning. I'm going to stay home today and see if I can get rid of it."

"I'm sorry, Mr. Hawksworth. I'll check your calendar and reschedule any appointments you might have. Take care of yourself. We'll look forward to seeing you tomorrow if you're feeling better."

Dana started to hang up. The exertion of talking had been almost more than he could handle.

"Oh, Mr. Hawksworth . . . Wait!"

"Yes, Helen?" Whatever it is, make it quick, he thought to himself, holding his head with his hand.

"Mr. Carter called me a few minutes ago and said he wanted to see you in his office just as soon as you arrived." Mr. Carter was the Executive Vice-President of the Lowery family's chain of stores and was Dana's immediate superior.

"Tell him I'm sick. I'll see him tomorrow." Dana put the phone back on the hook, sat down, and began sipping the glass of milk. He had to hold it with both hands to keep it from spilling.

"I've got to go back to bed before I drop," Dana told himself. He made his way into the living room, his head reeling. He managed to reach the couch, fell on it, and closed his eyes. "Let me sleep," he thought to himself. "Dear God, let me sleep."

But instead he tried once more to remember what he

had done to get himself in such a state. He recalled taking
his dinner break at 5:30. He knew he had been scheduled
to work until closing at 9 that night, but he couldn't remember returning to the store. In fact he couldn't remember anything until he awakened in bed a few minutes
ago.

"Maybe I didn't go back to the store," he thought. "I had
some appointments with customers. Maybe I missed them.
That could be why Mr. Carter wanted to see me.

"If that's all it is, it won't be much trouble. I can reschedule the customers and tell Mr. Carter some excuse or
other he'll believe."

The lies again. Every time he had one of the blackouts
he swore that the lies necessary to get himself off the hook
would be his last. In the future there would be no more
blackouts and no more dishonesty. But things never
worked out that way. He kept having periods he couldn't
remember, periods when he had to find excuses for having
done the unforgivable. It was a crazy way to live . . . Crazy
. . . Dana wondered if he *was* in full possession of his
mind.

He began drifting to sleep. There was a sound. It
started, then stopped, then started again. He cursed its
persistence.

Dana's eyes opened. The telephone. The sound was the
ringing telephone. He decided not to answer it, counting
the rings to see how many there would be before it quit.
Eight rings . . . nine rings . . . Still it continued. Fifteen
rings . . . Eighteen rings . . . Whoever it was wasn't going
to stop.

"It must be Ann," thought Dana. If she was trying to get
hold of him she would keep ringing like that. She knew he
had been in bed when she left. She'd wait until he awakened sufficiently to pick up the receiver.

Dana inched back to the telephone. "Hello?"

"I see you're still at home," said Ann. Her voice was formal. She was obviously angry. She had been through this
with him too often. Once she would have listened to his

excuses but now she knew they were lies and she was tired of hearing them.

"I called in sick. I feel terrible."

"What in hell did you do last night?"

"Just had too much to drink, I guess. I told Helen I had the flu, though."

"Have you seen your car yet?"

"No. Why?"

"The whole side is smashed in. The front wheel's so bent it's a miracle you ever drove it home. I don't even think it can be repaired. It looks like a total wreck."

Her voice had a hard edge to it, a fact that hurt Dana far more than the hangover. She was a soft, gentle woman who had always been slow to anger and quick to forgive. It took a great deal to make her upset, and now she was obviously furious.

"Are you going to be home when I get there?" she asked.

"Sure. Why not?"

"I never know where you'll be half the time. You ought to know that by now." She hung up.

Dana forced himself to check the car. He was certain Ann had been exaggerating; nobody could do as much damage as she claimed and not remember it. Perhaps it was just a small dent, picked up in a parking lot somewhere.

"Oh, my God!" he said when he saw the vehicle. Ann hadn't exaggerated in the least. The reality, if anything, was even worse than she had stated. He'd have to think of some excuse to tell her but he didn't know what. How can you lie about what caused an accident when you've never been in one? Dana had awakened at crash scenes often enough, of course, but he had never actually had an accident himself. Anyway, he couldn't remember having had one.

Dana went back inside the house and poured himself another glass of milk. The phone rang before he could drink it.

"Dana?" said the voice on the line. It had the unmistakable inflection of a New Yorker. Dana recognized it at once.

"Yes, Mr. Carter?" There was no reason for the man to bother him at home when he had called in sick. No reason at all—he hoped.

"How do you feel?"

"Lousy, Sir."

"Sorry to hear that, but I can understand why. I have to talk to you about last night." He was speaking slowly. It was obvious he was choosing his words carefully. "How soon can you get to the store?"

"I can't, Sir. I wrecked my car last night. I don't have any transportation." Dana was certain now that something had happened at the furniture store during his blackout. He didn't know what but it must have been serious and he must have been partly responsible.

"That's too bad. Please wait a moment." The phone clicked as though it had been put on "hold."

"Dana? This is Beth." The voice that came on the line was that of the President's wife. He had worked with her a few times in the past. They had always gotten along well.

"Hello, Mrs. Lowery."

"I want to talk with you as one friend to another. Where can you meet me? I understand about your car but I'll drive to your town. It's quite important."

Dana named a small restaurant a few miles from the house. He owned an aged, battered truck that barely ran but it would get him there and back without difficulty.

"It's a forty-five-minute drive from where you are now," Dana told her.

"That's all right. I'll leave immediately."

Dana was frightened when he hung up the phone. There was no reason for everyone to act so mysteriously. Surely whatever had happened could be discussed over the telephone. Yet Mrs. Lowery was coming to meet with him personally. It made no sense. If he could only remember. . . .

He went into the bathroom to shave and try to make himself look presentable. He had the appearance of the "Before" person on an antacid commercial. Washing his face and combing his hair did little to improve things. Still, he was supposed to be suffering from the flu, not making a favorable impression.

Dana met Beth Lowery as planned. He normally found it quite easy to talk with her but this time his mouth was dry and he had difficulty speaking.

"I hear you had quite a night," said Beth, forcing a smile. She was thirty-five years old, with the appearance and figure of a model, despite having two children and a strong hand in the business.

Dana and Beth had a mutual respect for each other. He suspected that it was this respect that had made her want to meet him like this—to give him another chance. But what had he done?

"Dana, I've worked with you for almost a year. My husband and Mr. Carter have been impressed with your basic abilities and your coolness under stress." The speech had obviously been rehearsed on the drive over. She paused, let out her breath, then said, "What happened last night? What caused you to become so violent and destructive? It just wasn't like you."

"I'm sorry, Beth. Things must have just gotten to me." He didn't know what she was talking about.

"You've always been so consistently steady. Frank was especially shocked by your conduct. He has forgiven you, though. In fact, if someone else hadn't witnessed what went on, we never would have known about it. Frank was reluctant to talk about it. He has so much respect for you he didn't want to hurt you by discussing what happened."

"I'm very sorry, Beth. I don't know what got into me. It's never happened before."

"You must have been wound up inside. The business pressures must have been eating away at you. Why don't you take the rest of the week off? You know you're one of the most rational people any of us ever met. That's why your actions are so shocking. The people who saw you thought you acted almost insane."

"I've had a lot of personal problems. Getting time off

will help me get on top of them. I'll call Frank and tell
him how sorry I am."

Dana left the restaurant with relief. He still had his job,
but whatever had happened must have been terrible. It
was only later that he learned the truth.

Ann was cold and angry when she returned home that
evening. She had reached the limits of her endurance. "I
don't think I care what you do any more," she told him.
"From the looks of the car, one day you'll kill yourself and
then I won't have to worry anymore. But what you're doing to me doesn't matter. The kids have reached an age
when they know a little of what's going on. They're the
ones you're hurting."

There was nothing for Dana to say. Ann would stand by
him as she always had. Yet life, he knew, would never be
what he had once expected. Something inside his head
made him his own worst enemy and he didn't know how to
deal with it. He wanted to be like everyone else, to stop
causing so much sorrow for those he loved, but he didn't
know how to do it. He didn't even know when he did those
things people told him about.

Then one day a short while later, Ann was sitting in the
living room reading a copy of *Science Digest*, to which
Dana subscribed. "Dana?" she called excitedly. "Come
here. I've got something to show you."

It was an article about the use of Lithium in the treatment of people with manic-depressive problems. According to the article, many of those treated with the drug
were able to lead completely normal lives. "Do you think it
might help you?" she asked. "Those doctors you've consulted in the past have said you're manic-depressive."

By this time Dana was ready to try anything. He immediately called the family doctor and asked him for the
names of psychiatrists in the area who were using Lithium
in the treatment of their manic-depressive patients.

The family doctor was enthusiastic. He knew about Dana's mental problems. He also had another patient diagnosed as manic-depressive, a woman who was being

treated with Lithium and was leading a normal life. He warned Dana, however, that the drug had serious side effects and required frequent blood tests to keep track of them. He gave Dana the names of three psychiatrists who he knew were using the drug as one of their treatment tools.

Dana excitedly dialed the telephone number of the first psychiatrist on the list. His line was busy and Dana was too impatient to wait for whoever was talking to hang up. He dialed the number of the second name he had been given and was pleased when he heard the telephone at the other end of the line start ringing.

"Dr. Ralph Allison's office," a woman's voice said. Dana told her his problem and she set up a time when he could come to Santa Cruz for a visit with the psychiatrist.

Dana didn't know it, but his lifelong nightmare was about to come to an end.

CHAPTER 20

It was March 30, 1975, an unusually warm day for the time of year. Dana wondered whether there would be a hot summer as he left his car and headed for the modern one-story building in which Dr. Ralph Allison's office was located.

He was somewhat apprehensive as he went inside. It wasn't the idea of exposing his life to a psychiatrist that bothered him. Rather it was a concern about whether this doctor would be able to provide some answers to his problems. Perhaps if the Lithium modified his behavior enough, Ann would stay with him. He knew she couldn't take living with his erratic behavior much longer.

"The doctor's expecting you," said the receptionist, smiling. She was friendly, putting him at ease. Dana thought she would probably be very good in sales.

There were two doors between the waiting area and the doctor's own office. Apparently they were meant to slow the flight of anyone who suddenly became violent.

The room where the doctor met Dana was dominated by

a walnut desk and large padded chair. There was a file cabinet to one side of the entrance and a small bookcase filled with books along the back wall. Another chair, thickly padded in brown tweed and designed for reclining, was where the patients sat. A matching sofa in the same brown tweed stood against another wall.

Dr. Allison was a tall, middle-aged man with dark hair and glasses. His face remained impassive while Dana spoke, though Dana sensed that the blank expression was the result of training rather than a lack of compassion.

Dana told him that he had been referred by his family physician because of his drinking problem and the manic-depressive diagnosis. He discussed his apparent actions during drinking bouts and his attempt to work with Alcoholics Anonymous. He avoided going into detail about the memory lapses, though. He was not yet ready to reveal what were, to him, the more frightening aspects of his problem.

Based on what Dana told him, Dr. Allison confirmed the manic-depressive diagnosis and agreed to try Lithium therapy. He prescribed a minimal dosage and arranged for the first of the blood tests that would be necessary while he was receiving the medication.

Dana was barely into the therapy when Johnny once again created havoc at Lowery's furniture store. This time there would be no forgiveness; no second chance. He was fired on the spot—a fact that delighted Johnny.

Though the incident upset Dana, he was able to go job hunting once more with the thought that it might be for the last time. He felt that as he advanced in Lithium therapy he would at last gain control and be able to live a normal life.

The next few weeks passed without serious incident. He was experiencing mild side effects from the Lithium, primarily a shakiness that caused him to spill his coffee, but nothing so severe that he had to stop taking it. Even Ann felt there was a chance for a normal life again.

Ann had family in Canada and had wanted for some

time to go north for a brief vacation. At last she felt Dana
could get along without her so she and the two boys made
plans for the trip. Dana was working another new job and
couldn't arrange for time off. Linda, who had a summer
job, also would stay home.

Then, three days before Ann's scheduled departure,
Dana once more failed to return from work. Ann was
crushed. She had put her faith in the Lithium therapy and
now she realized that it was almost certainly not working.
There would be no miracles. From what she had read,
Ann knew that Lithium was the only hope a manic-
depressive had of being able to lead a normal life. If it
didn't work, probably nothing would.

There was, she realized, no future with Dana. Whatever
joy life had in store for her would have to be hers alone.
She loved the side of Dana that was devoted to the family,
but that alone wasn't enough to make her want to put up
with the violence and the trips to Reno and Las Vegas,
where she was certain he was seeing other women, any
longer. She couldn't continue to be married to half a husband. She decided to take the boys and go to Canada as
planned. All that would change would be the return trip.
If life in Canada with her family seemed potentially rewarding, she decided she would not come back ever again.

It was three in the morning when Dana finally called.
He had lost his car, and sheepishly asked if she could come
to get him. Once again she drove out to rescue him, knowing in her heart that it would probably be for the last
time.

The ride home was in silence. Ann didn't ask Dana
where he had been or how he had lost the car. If he knew,
he probably wouldn't tell her. And if he didn't know, he
probably would lie to cover the fact. Canada was still the
only answer.

Dana also felt his life had ended. During the ride home
he searched his mind for an explanation of what had happened that night. The blackouts had returned. He had
found himself in an all-night coffee shop, liquor on his

breath, with no knowledge of what he had been doing prior to the time he was sitting there. He had searched the parking lot and nearby streets for the car without success.

Dana wondered why he even bothered to go on. He loved his wife and children but how much longer could they put up with him? He didn't know Ann's thoughts concerning Canada, but they would not have surprised him.

Two days later Ann and the boys left as planned. Dana still was without his car, despite having searched every bar parking lot anywhere near the coffee shop. He finally reported it stolen and hoped the police might locate it.

That Sunday morning Dana borrowed his daughter's car to drive to a nearby market and buy a newspaper. As he pulled out of the drive, the depression hit him once more and he was aware of nothing more until Monday morning when he awakened in a motel room. The address was thirty miles from his home and Linda's car, too, was missing. Dana didn't know what he had done with it or why he had gone to the motel.

He dressed and hitch-hiked home. When he arrived he called Linda, who had managed to get a friend to take her to work. She was furious with him.

She arrived home two hours later, driving a borrowed car. Her temper was just barely under control. She informed her father coldly that they were going to look for her car until they found it, no matter how long it took.

The search began at the motel. From there they began driving in an ever-widening circle until, three hours later, they spotted it. The car was well hidden in a clump of trees about a half mile from the motel. Apparently Johnny had decided that he could cause Dana extra pain by leaving his car in so illogical a location that it would be difficult for him to find it. Not only would the loss of the car upset Dana, it would also further disrupt his strained home life.

Dana had an appointment with Dr. Allison the following day. He was hesitant to admit the Lithium might not be working, yet he knew he had to tell the truth. There was no way the doctor could help him with his problem unless he was perfectly honest with him. During the previous sessions he had begun admitting to the blackouts; this was just one more piece of the puzzle that seemed to be without solution.

The doctor was silent after hearing the story of the last several days. Finally he said, "Let's dig a little into your subconscious and see if we can find what's been happening."

Dana wasn't certain what to expect, but after all he had been through he was willing to try anything.

"Lie back in your chair," said Dr. Allison. "I want you to relax; to make yourself as comfortable as you can."

Dana did as he was told. His heart was beating rapidly. He summoned all his will power, trying to force himself to be calm. He kept telling himself this might bring about the answer he had been seeking.

"Now close your eyes."

Dana complied. Then he began counting backwards from ten. The doctor was using his training in hypnosis to put Dana into a sleeplike state. It was a standard therapeutic tool, which he had used successfully many times in the past.

"Why did you go and get drunk?" asked the doctor. His voice seemed to be coming from a great distance. Dana heard it only faintly.

"Why did you go and get drunk?" the doctor repeated.

Dana failed to answer.

The doctor had Dana relax more fully, taking him deeper into hypnosis. He repeated the question, but still Dana did not respond. No answer had formed in his mind.

Dr. Allison waited a moment, hoping Dana would say something. When it became obvious that nothing would be brought forth even by hypnosis, he decided to return Dana to full wakefulness. He told him to begin counting forward. One . . . Two . . . Three. . . .

Dana opened his eyes and said, "I don't drink. Johnny does." The words startled him. He didn't know why he had said them or what they meant.

"Who is Johnny?" asked Dr. Allison. His face retained its

familiar lack of expression but his body was suddenly
tense. He was obviously as surprised by the statement as
Dana had been.

"I don't know why I said that, Doctor," said Dana. He
was confused by the words and what they might mean.

"Who is Johnny?" the doctor repeated.

Dana felt foolish. He realized that the doctor was going
to keep asking him that question until he came up with an
answer. But the only Johnny he knew had been an imaginary playmate back when he was a child. It seemed silly
to mention that to the doctor. It had been so long ago and
he had long since put it from his mind.

"All I can think of is that I had an imaginary playmate
named Johnny when I was a small boy," said Dana, sheepishly. "But what would that have to do with my problem?"

"Maybe nothing, Dana. But it could have meaning.
You've had blackouts and behavior changes. The fact that
you had an imaginary playmate could lead to a diagnosis
quite different from the manic-depressive state we assumed was your problem. You have many of the symptoms
of what is known as multiple personality."

Suddenly the movie Dana and Ann had seen so many
years earlier came back to his memory. "You mean like
The Three Faces of Eve or a Dr. Jekyll and Mr. Hyde?" As
he said the words he realized that Ann had often used the
Jekyll and Hyde adjectives to describe behavior he
couldn't remember.

Dana's mind drifted back over the years. He remembered the poetry he had found. He remembered hearing
accounts of his own bizarre behavior, behavior he knew
nothing about. He remembered the countless blackouts
during which he supposedly did things that went against
his basic character. Multiple personality?

"This isn't my final diagnosis," said the doctor. "You may
not be a multiple personality. It's just one of the possibilities I feel should be considered.

"Now tell me what you remember about Johnny."

Dana remembered almost nothing about Johnny except

that he had been an imaginary playmate, so he related what he had been told about him by family members. He had put that aspect of his childhood from his mind many years ago.

The hour ended with nothing resolved. Yet the idea of being a multiple personality wouldn't leave his mind. Exactly what did multiple personality mean? Was he two people? Or possessed by the devil? It seemed ridiculous.

Yet somehow, when he didn't let his imagination run away with him, having more than one personality made sense. People had told him he was childlike at times. Others had called him a wild man. Everyone who had known him for any length of time said he was changeable, yet he never actually remembered acting any other way than he normally did. The wild changes he was told about invariably took place during those periods when he was suffering from amnesia. Perhaps there really was more than one personality controlling him. In fact, thinking back on his behavior over the years, the multiple personality diagnosis was the first that might account for all aspects of his actions.

Dana discussed the possible diagnosis with his daughter as soon as he returned home. To his surprise, she was able to accept it at once. It made immediate sense to her. It explained everything that she had once thought was beyond explanation.

Ann telephoned from Canada the next day and Dana told her something new had developed in his therapy. He wanted to talk with her about it but felt he couldn't over the telephone. Something in his voice must have convinced her that there was new hope, for three days later she arrived back home with the boys.

She listened with great interest to the story of Johnny and the idea of a multiple personality, her mind meanwhile racing back over the years. She recalled the day of the picnic when Dana was still courting her. She remembered the poem shown to her by what she had thought was a childlike facet of Dana's own personality. She remembered other poems and other periods of change. She thought about the abusive language and sexual aggression of "Mr. Hyde." She remembered driving with Dana when he was calm, collected, and soberly traveling the highway within the speed limit, then suddenly seeing him hard and mean, his foot pressing the accelerator to the floor. What had once seemed his irrational "moods" suddenly had an explanation. She smiled and relaxed in her chair, the tensions of the last twenty years beginning to leave her body.

"There's no question in my mind that Johnny is real and that multiple personality is your problem," she said quietly. At last the illness had a label. There would be no more gray areas. Everything that had happened during the years of their marriage was readily explainable with this diagnosis, something that had not been the case when they had assumed, years earlier, that he was a manic-depressive.

Once again Ann had hope and this time she felt it would not be frustrated. Surely a psychiatrist who could recognize such a condition in Dana would also be able to cure it. What she didn't know at the time was that in order to effect that cure, her husband would have to die.

CHAPTER 21

During the next few months, Dana learned that being able to identify a problem is still a far cry from solving it. Despite all his and Dr. Allison's best intentions, it would be a long time before all the diverse pieces of my personality would be united into a single whole.

To begin with, several sessions were required before the various personalities could be identified and the diagnosis confirmed. Ann attended these sessions and later told Dana what had taken place during them. Through hypnosis the other personalities were called forth and photographed with a Polaroid camera so that Dana could view himself as others had seen him. The experience was a shock for him but it did help him to accept the reality of the problem that had plagued him for forty years.

At a session that took place on July 30, 1975, a fifth personality was discovered within my mind. This was Jerry. The only reason for his existence seemed to be to help the doctor assemble a healthy individual from the jigsaw puzzle he had encountered within me. Jerry's initial appearance was brief—just long enough to reveal his existence and to warn Dana not to drink because it would help Johnny take control.

About this time Dr. Allison began to use age regression in his treatment. Through hypnosis he would take Dana back in time to an age when one of the personalities was particularly active. Then he would find the reason for the personality's taking control and try to deal with it.

Dana learned that multiple personality is one way the mind has of coping with problems it can't handle in any other way. Dana was incapable of being angry so he had created Johnny, who was all anger, violence, and hate. He also was unable to express love so Peter handled such tender emotions.

Dana had always had trouble understanding his parents and what they expected of him. When an event occurred that was particularly upsetting for him, he would act out his emotions by letting another personality take control. The doctor was attempting to get Dana to face these events, to understand them and deal with them without switching personalities. He had found in the past that when the emotional traumas in the life of a multiple-personality patient are understood, the need for the additional personalities vanishes. The patient learns to handle future problems in a normal manner and is able to express a normal range of feeling.

Johnny, meanwhile, had become aware of what the doctor was trying to do for Dana and it frightened him. If Dana were cured there would no longer be any way Johnny could continue with his existence. He feared the therapy and the new personality, Jerry. Frequently Dana would be sitting with a pencil and piece of paper in front of him when Johnny would suddenly write him a message. Once, for example, Dana was in the doctor's office when his hand suddenly wrote: "Hi, bastard! Jerry is only half. I'll do you a favor. I'll get rid of him. He's no good. Bang! Bang! He's dead! Love, Johnny."

A session that took place on September 10, 1975, was

typical of Dana's treatment during this period. He had a 10 A.M. appointment with Dr. Allison that day. As he drove the several miles to the office he was thinking of the drugs he was still taking and how their physical side effects were frustrating his existence. He was constantly listless and the Lithium was producing shakes and muscle tremors.

The previous weekend had been especially upsetting. His mother-in-law had celebrated her seventy-third birthday and at the party he had tried to play catch with one of his sons. To his great disappointment the game had stopped almost as soon as it had started because he hadn't been able to control the ball when throwing it and hadn't had the dexterity to catch it. He had been unable to enjoy even so simple a pleasure as the game would have given him.

Moreover, he was beginning to find the treatment frustrating. He still wasn't cured and was beginning to think he never would be. He had lost three different jobs since the Lowery furniture chain had let him go, and Johnny had not given up his ability to take control. His marriage, moreover, was still far from idyllic and his children continued to question his erratic behavior.

"Hi, Dana, you're a little early," said the receptionist when he arrived in the psychiatrist's office. "How about a cup of coffee while waiting?"

"Sure—two sugars and no cream." He smiled, then frowned again when he discovered he could hold the cup only by grasping it with both hands. Even then he shook so badly that some of the hot liquid spilled over onto his wrist. The damned Lithium was affecting him again.

The session began as it always did. He sat on the reclining chair and the doctor took a chair opposite him. As usual the doctor's face contained no hint of expression. It had become a game for Dana to try and read something in his eyes and mouth, some sign that his own emotions were having an effect on the psychiatrist. He never could, though over the many weeks of treatment he had learned that the doctor had great empathy for his patients. He was a warm, caring individual and the mask he made of his face was strictly professional.

"How have you been doing this past week?" asked the doctor.

"All right, I guess, Doctor," Dana lied. There was no reply, so he continued. "Actually, these drugs are driving me up a tree. Between the shakes and the listlessness I find myself struggling at about half steam at work."

Dana paused, waiting for the doctor to say something. He was greeted by silence.

"The shakes have added a new dimension to my love-making, too. That is, if I don't fall asleep from the other medication before I even get started. When I do fall asleep my relation with Ann has deteriorated to the point where she doesn't bother awakening me. We only attempt to do it on Saturday night as it is. Any other time I'm rejected. So if I'm unlucky enough to be put to sleep by the medicine on Saturday, it's a whole week before I can try again. Maybe I should skip all the pills on Saturday."

"Do you think that's what you should do?" asked the doctor.

"No. I guess not. But I'm getting tired of taking those pills, that's for certain!"

"Have you heard from Johnny this week?"

"No, but I've had a slight depression all week. It's not as bad as the one I get just before he takes over, but it seems like he wants to come out. Maybe the pills are holding him back."

"That's why I'm having you take them. Have you tried a two-way conversation with Phil or Jerry this week?" The doctor had shown Dana that through self-hypnosis it was possible for him to hold conversations with either of the two personalities who tried to help him during bad times. Phil had always rescued him from harm. Jerry's purpose was to help him unite the personalities into one whole, normal individual.

"Yes, Doctor, I tried, but I feel dumb sitting in the dark talking to myself. And this last week it hasn't worked very well, either. I guess I've been in the wrong frame of mind for such things."

Dana was feeling sorry for himself. Dr. Allison recognized the problem and suggested they begin the therapy session. He took some typing paper and placed it in front of Dana, who sat up and took a pencil in his hand. He was going to use automatic writing.

Automatic writing is a tool widely accepted by psychologists and psychiatrists. They have found that some people will write thoughts that are quite different from what is going through their conscious minds. It is a way of reaching the unconscious—which, in Dana's case, meant reaching Phil and/or Jerry.

Dr. Allison watched Dana hold the pen. He began gently stroking Dana's writing arm while telling him to relax. He then said anyone inside Dana's mind who wanted to say something should write. Dana closed his eyes and lost consciousness for a moment. When he awakened he saw the scrawled message:

"You need me. Let me out soon before it is too late. This experiment is a lot of damned foolishness. Let things stay the way they've always been. It's much simpler. Okay?" It was signed by Johnny.

Dana had been through this experience several times by now, yet seeing messages on the paper in handwriting other than his own always shocked him.

Dr. Allison read the message, then said, "Dana, last week you asked me why Johnny would burn your arms with cigarettes over the years. I gave you an answer, but I think we should ask him personally since he's trying to talk with us through the automatic writing."

Dr. Allison handed Dana a fresh sheet of paper. "Write across the top the question, 'Why have my arms been burned with cigarettes?' "

Dana followed his instructions. Then he closed his eyes and briefly lost consciousness. He awoke to find the answer, "It's my way of saying 'Fuck you!' Bye, Johnny."

The doctor took the sheets of paper and placed them in

his file. Then he had Dana sit on the recliner. "Okay, Dana, sit back in your chair and relax. Close your eyes. I am going to count backward over the years until you have returned to age eleven."

Dana closed his eyes and relaxed as he had done many times before. He had been nervous about the use of hypnosis at first, but he was quite confortable with it now.

The doctor started counting. "Forty-two, forty-one, forty. . . . " The years rolled backwards. "You are now eleven years old. You are now eleven years old. Will the eleven-year-old Dana please come forward? I want to speak to the eleven-year-old Dana."

Dana's eyes popped open. His facial expressions and movements were those of a boy on the edge of adolescence. His voice was high-pitched when he spoke; as an eleven-year-old's, it had yet to change.

"Hi, Dana, how are you?" said Dr. Allison, smiling.

"Fine, Doctor," said Dana. "I remember you. You're a doctor and we've talked before."

"Almost a year ago, Dana." The doctor was referring to an earlier age regression session.

Dana looked about the room. It was all quite familiar to him. "Yes, I guess it was last year when I was ten that I was here. I don't remember coming here to see you today, though, but I forget things."

"How have things been going for you?"

"Okay."

"Have you been bothered by Johnny lately?"

"You mean my make-believe playmate I had when I was a child? Don't be silly!" Dana was fidgeting in his seat. The doctor's question upset him and he wished he could leave. But the doctor was a big person and it wouldn't be polite to go. He wondered where his mother was. He wished she'd come and take him home.

"Are you still being blamed for things you didn't do?" asked the doctor.

"Yes. Sometimes, Sir. I told you about that before."

"Yes, Dana, we have talked about this before. Tell me

about an incident that you got blamed for. Something you didn't do."

Dana thought a moment. "Well, Doctor, two weeks ago they said I shot the kid that lives down the block in the head with an arrow. It was in his backyard and he had to have stitches. But I wasn't even there. I told them I wasn't there and I told my mother I wasn't there. But they all told me I was lying."

"You shot the boy?"

"I don't know what happened. But I didn't shoot him!"

"It must have been someone who looked like you."

"Yes, Sir." Dana looked a little relieved.

"Could it be Johnny?"

Dana didn't answer him. The doctor waited a few moments, then said, "What else has happened to you since I talked to you last?"

"Oh, nothing much."

"What about your mother and father?"

"They yell a lot at night when they think I'm in bed a-sleep. My mother laughs and cries." He paused, then added, "I don't like school. The kids and teachers don't like me, but I don't care."

"Tell me about your mother and father. Why do they fight?"

"Cause my mother doesn't love my dad."

"That's most likely not true, Dana. You said your mother laughs and cries a lot. Sometimes crying and laughing can be symptoms of sickness. Your mother most likely is ill."

"I kind of remember something. I think someone else told me that about her and it made me feel better. I hope she gets well."

"Can you remember who else told you she was sick?"

"No, Sir."

"Do you remember when you were told it?"

"No, Sir. . . . " He paused. "Wait a minute. I remember it happened one night. My mother and father were fighting and I got out of bed and sneaked down to the basement where I couldn't hear them. I don't know how long I was there but I heard a voice say, 'Don't blame Mother. She's sick.' Or something like that. I looked around and nobody was there. But I did feel better. I went back to bed. Mom and Dad had stopped fighting and I went to sleep."

Dana began to feel dizzy. He started to sit up as the doctor said, "Whoever is responsible for Dana's feeling better that night, come out!" His voice was firm and commanding.

Dana closed his eyes, then opened them and sat up in the chair. His feet were firmly planted on the ground, his face more mature. Phil was in control.

"Hi, Doc."

"Hello, Phil. I thought it was probably you."

"Yeah, it was me. You know, 'Do-a-good-deed Phil.' "

"Phil, do you remember that far back?"

"Sure I do."

"How old are you?"

"A couple of years younger than Dana."

"Tell me, Phil, what was going on back there?"

"Well, Dana had everybody against him. That son-of-a-bitch Johnny was constantly getting him into all kinds of trouble. His dad was hassling him, his teachers thought he was strange, and the kids were leery of him."

"Phil, what could you do to help?"

Phil shifted his position in the chair, leaned forward, and said, "Doc, I wasn't as strong then as I am now. I would try to push that son-of-a-bitch Johnny aside as often as I could so Dana would have control. But I wasn't always successful. Then sometimes I would try to give Dana advice, though I was careful about it. I didn't want him to think he was going crazy from hearing voices and all."

Dr. Allison rose from his chair. "I'd like to take your photograph. Do you mind if I do it, Phil?"

"Hell, no! Go right ahead!"

Dr. Allison used a Polaroid camera to snap a picture of Phil. Phil smiled and posed a little. The smile faded after the flash and he said, "Doc, I know that I don't really have a body all to myself and I know that you are trying to cure Dana of Johnny. That's something I've been trying to do for years. But what happens to me when Dana's cured? Lately that has me kind of worried." He sat still, his body slightly tense as he waited for an answer.

Dr. Allison spoke slowly, carefully weighing his words. "Phil, your existence will change in a sense. I can't explain exactly how, but you and Peter will definitely survive."

"Thanks, Doc. I'll tell Peter. He's even more scared than I am. But he trusts you and it'll make him feel better to know what you said."

Phil closed his eyes and slumped in the chair. Dr. Allison called, "Dana. Dana."

"You fucking bastard!" said Johnny. The doctor's attempt to bring Dana back had been in vain. The man sitting in front of him was glaring. The hatred in his eyes was intense. "You can't beat me. I'm stronger than Dana and Phil and Peter and I sure as hell am stronger than you are."

"You're a nobody," said the doctor. "And you're already losing the battle."

Johnny angrily rose from the couch, glaring at his watch. "I'm not going to listen to this bullshit. I'm going out for a drink!" He started for the door.

But before he could get very far, Dr. Allison moved swiftly from his chair and struck him lightly on the forehead, between his eyes, with the open part of his palm. It was a technique discovered by a Swedish doctor and it always forced whatever personality was in control of the body at the time to submerge. A moment after he struck the blow, the doctor heard Dana say, "How did I do, Dr. Allison?" He was out of the hypnosis and no longer a child.

"It went well. I took a picture of Phil for you to see. I missed him during my last picture session."

Dana studied the face in the photograph. It was more expressive than his own but still quite similar. He had come to accept his multiple personality condition but was still bothered by the sight of one of his other selves. He returned the photograph to the doctor, who placed it in his files.

The session was over. They would meet again next week.

CHAPTER 22

The weeks quickly turned into months. During each session the doctor would probe more deeply into Dana's past. Using hypnosis to take Dana back to his childhood, he would uncover the problems he had faced and then discuss them with Dana so he would have a clearer understanding of himself and his family.

During all these sessions Dr. Allison had been working on the assumption that Peter, Phil, Johnny, and Jerry were all fragments of Dana's mind. But then on November 12, 1975, there suddenly appeared a hint that this theory might be wrong. While Jerry was speaking through the use of automatic writing, the name Henry came up for the first time.

"Who is Henry?" asked Dr. Allison. Dana had also been surprised to see the name on the paper.

"Henry's my real first name. I'm legally Henry Dana Hawksworth but I've always used the name Dana. I guess I must have subconsciously reverted to my original name."

Nothing further was said.

During this therapy period Johnny was making his last efforts to raise hell. The first occasion was in March. Dana was working in the appliance department of a major department store. The store was open until nine that night and Dana had the late shift.

Shortly before five Dana left for his dinner break, walking to a nearby drugstore to buy a pair of sunglasses. He entered the store quietly, his face empty of expression as he walked to the display rack. The clerk gave him only a passing glance, then went back to looking through the evening paper.

Dana rejected the first two pairs of sunglasses as being the wrong styles for his taste. As he started to take down a third pair, the depression struck. A moment later Johnny was standing before the mirror.

Johnny's lip curled upward, his eyes narrowed, and his expression hardened. He put the glasses back on the rack, turned, and walked heavily toward the door. He swaggered past the sales clerk, making an obscene comment to her as he passed.

Johnny knew Dana was expected back at the store but he didn't care. That chickenshit was a sucker—one of those jerks who thinks the way to get along in life is with a steady job, a wife, and kids. But Johnny knew better. He headed toward his favorite bar, laughing to himself about the trouble Dana would have when his boss discovered he hadn't returned from his break.

It was seven o'clock in the evening when he finally left the bar and headed for Dana's car. The night air was cool and Johnny thought the evening perfect for driving. He turned the key in the ignition, then put the gas pedal to the floor. The small foreign car pulled screeching from the curb, accelerating rapidly.

Johnny began weaving in and out of traffic, racing lights and narrowly missing oncoming cars. He came to a sharp corner, down-shifted, and spun the wheel. The liquor had affected his timing, though. The car struck the curb with such force that the right front tire was torn off the car, leaving only the rim.

"To hell with it," thought Johnny after recovering from the jolt. "It's not my car! Let Dana worry about getting it fixed. I'm going to keep driving."

Once again the car picked up speed, though not quite as rapidly as before. Johnny was fighting the steering wheel in an effort to make the lopsided vehicle continue on a relatively straight path. Sparks were flying as the rim jarred against the pavement and several passing motorists sounded their horns to signal him that his tire was gone. He ignored them.

Johnny turned another corner and drove past a police cruiser on a routine patrol. The officer was surprised to see the damaged car traveling so rapidly. He thought something must be wrong so he turned on his lights and siren, made a U-turn, and took off in pursuit.

"Stupid pig!" thought Johnny, glancing in his rear-view mirror. If the car hadn't been damaged he would have tried to outrun the policeman. But that was impossible, so he did the only thing he could do. He pulled over to the curb and stopped the car.

"Are you aware you're driving without one tire?" asked the police officer. He could tell Johnny had been drinking.

Of course he was aware. Did the pig think he was too drunk to know his tire was gone? Well, two could play this stupid game. "I'm not missing any tires," Johnny told him.

The officer asked him to step from the car and take a look at the disabled vehicle. Johnny walked over to where the rim was against the ground, stooped down, and said, "What did I tell you? All four tires are in perfect shape. This one even has most of the tread left."

The officer placed Johnny in the cruiser and took him to the police station for a chemical test to determine how much alcohol was in his body.

As soon as the technician was ready to start the test, Johnny became defiant. "I won't take the chemical test.

You'll have to use some other method," he told them.

"Would you agree to a urine analysis?" the technician asked. Johnny said he would. However, when this had been readied he said he had changed his mind. They would have to give him a breath test.

Once again the technician changed his equipment. Johnny watched with amusement as he went to all the trouble of getting set up. Then he stated, "I've changed my mind again. I'm not taking any of your damned tests!"

"Then we're going to have to put you in jail," said the police officer. He led Johnny down the hall to the cell area.

Johnny was disgusted when he saw the drunk tank. Some of its occupants had vomited, then passed out before they could be cleaned up. Others were too drunk to go to the toilet and were sitting in urine-stained pants. The noise and the smells formed a nauseating mixture. Johnny decided to turn the body back to Dana and let him "enjoy" the atmosphere on his own.

Ann rescued Dana from the jail, furious over this latest in a long line of Johnny's "incidents." She knew Dana was innocent, but that didn't make the affair easier to take. They both wondered if their faith in the psychiatrist had been misplaced.

Dana didn't lose his job over the drunk-driving incident. He was away from the store only a few hours and he was forgiven. Johnny was infuriated by all this, of course. He was determined to get Dana fired.

His next opportunity came just a short while later. Dana was in a bar near the store, having a drink with Larry, a salesman in the men's clothing department. Suddenly Johnny took control, grabbing a candle holder on the counter and shattering it against the bar. "I'm going to smash you the same way," he said. Larry tried to calm him down, but Johnny struck him, sending the 250-pound clothing salesman sprawling on the floor.

Johnny rose from his stool, his eyes blazing. He was going to show that fat-assed son-of-a-bitch to mind his own business. As Larry struggled to get up, Johnny drew his foot back to kick him in the face.

One of the other patrons had been watching Johnny's explosion and realized that the kick might kill the fallen man. In the nick of time he knocked Johnny off balance, causing him to miss the blow.

Johnny regained his footing, turned, and slammed his elbow into the bystander who had pushed him. The man doubled over and Johnny hit him again.

Meanwhile Larry had gotten to his feet and realized he had better run before Johnny turned on him again. He reached the store and raced up the steps to his department.

Johnny followed him into the store, moving slowly, deliberately. His rage was barely contained. He walked to the elevator, people moving away from him as he approached. He didn't say or do anything to those he passed, but they could sense the hostility in him.

Johnny had lost interest in Larry. Instead of pursuing him to the men's clothing section, he went to the appliance department where Dana worked. He picked up a 19-inch television set and heaved it across the room. Then he walked over to a desk where the department head had left some papers from a big sale he had made. Johnny tore the papers into shreds, then left the store for another round of drinking.

The next morning was Saturday and Dana awakened at 7:30 A.M. He had no memory of the night before, though his head throbbed with a hangover.

He was depressed by the certain knowledge that Johnny had again been in control. His therapy had brought him an understanding of his illness and the emotional traumas that had led a normal mind to fragment. Yet understanding had not brought the fusion of the personalities into one. He still was not cured.

He rose from the bed and walked into the bathroom to shave. He wondered what time he had returned home the night before. Ann normally told him when he had come in but she and Linda were away for the weekend. His sons were in the house, but they had almost certainly been asleep when he had come home.

He went into the kitchen to get some coffee and orange
juice. His sons joined him. Mark commented that Dana's
boss had called from the department store. He had been
concerned with the way Dana had behaved the day before.
He had told Mark about his father's violent eruption and
said he was worried about Dana's mind.

The news shocked Dana. This was one job he desperately
wanted to retain, yet he knew he would not be able to any
longer. No one would risk keeping him on after what
Johnny had obviously done. He was sad and depressed,
hating himself, his illness, and his life. He told his sons,
however, that he felt the report was undoubtedly an exaggeration.

Dana left the house and began the long drive to work.
After he had gone ten miles a wave of depression came
over him. Knowing what that might mean, he summoned
all his will to fight another personality taking over. He
pulled to the side of the road and concentrated on staying
in control. After a few moments the feeling passed, though
he remained saddened by yet another reminder of his illness.

As he tried to compose himself, he looked around the
area. He was on a mountain road, just five feet away from
a drop-off that was almost 500 feet straight down. He realized that all he had to do was drive six feet more and he,
the car, and Johnny would all be destroyed. There would
be no more alter-personalities taking over; no more embarrassment and shame for Ann; no more awakening in
strange places without any knowledge of where he was or
how he had gotten there.

He restarted the engine and released the brake, then
turned the wheel so the car was aimed for the cliff. Slowly
he pressed his foot against the accelerator. The tires spun
on the gravel, then gripped and pulled the car rapidly
towards the edge.

"That was close!" thought Phil, wrenching the wheel
back to the left and returning the car to the road.
"Another second and we'd have been done for."

Phil turned the car around and drove back to Dana's house, surprising Scott and Mark, who had not expected him home for several hours. "I'm going to call Dr. Allison," Phil explained. "I have to admit myself to the Dominican Hospital's Crisis Intervention Ward."

"Do you want me to drive you, Dad?" asked Mark. He was home on leave from the Navy.

"That won't be necessary," said Phil. "I'm in full control." He called Dr. Allison, leaving word with the doctor's answering service that Dana was going to Dominican Hospital.

"I'm Dr. Allison's patient," Phil told the receptionist when he reached the hospital. "I'm a potential suicide and need to be admitted at once."

The receptionist stared at him. His voice was calm and controlled, unlike that of most suicidal patients. He had not told her that it was actually Dana who wanted to take his life, not Phil. He knew that would only confuse her and delay the admission procedure.

"Dr. Allison called shortly before you arrived," said the receptionist. "He said to expect you."

A few moments later a nurse from the Crisis Intervention Ward came to care for him. She was also surprised by Phil's appearance. He looked more like a doctor or a pharmaceutical company salesman making a business call than a potential suicide.

The nurse took Phil to an examining room just as Dr. Allison arrived. Phil gave the doctor a rundown on what had happened, still not identifying himself. The doctor, however, suspected he was Phil, and was about to ask him whether he was when Dana again took control of the body.

Dana showed no emotion upon learning where he was. His only regret was that his suicide attempt had failed. He was assigned to one of the small rooms occupied by the patients during the short time they were in the hospital. The rooms were typical single-bed rooms except that they lacked telephones and television sets. The lack of telephones insured the patients freedom from family and other outside pressures. The lack of television sets forced the patients to go for diversion to the large open area at the end of the hall where they would mix with one another. A television set, ping-pong table, writing desk, and other recreational items were located there.

Dana was exhausted when he reached his room. He slept soundly for the next three hours.

On April 25, 1976, he began keeping a journal of his hospital stay. Dr. Allison was giving him intense therapy to resolve the last few conflicts in his life. If all went well, the doctor had told him, the separate personalities should soon fuse into the original Henry. If all went well. . . .

"*I feel out of place,*" Dana wrote in his journal that day. "*I know why I'm here. I checked myself in because I was afraid I might kill myself or change into Johnny and create more havoc.*

"*Why is Johnny trying to destroy me? He owes me his life, yet he is trying to take mine. All of my life I have been haunted by the two sides of one coin. My own Jekyll and Hyde—Dana and Johnny, as well as Peter and Phil to complicate things. Why is this?*

"*Again I ask why I'm here. Am I so different? Johnny is not me. Yet he wears my body and ruins my world. Why can't he die and I live? Maybe death will destroy him and I can come back and start all over again.*

"*Or maybe it doesn't work that way. Maybe he comes back and starts all over again without me. He has no soul; he can't come back. Maybe I don't have a soul either. Should I give up? Should I surrender to Johnny? It would be an easy way to die. Just go away and let Johnny have it all. I'm tired of the fight, so tired.*

"*But I can't quit. That's why I'm here. The last big battle and Johnny is going to lose. Dr. Allison is the General, the nurse is his Major, and I'm the Lieutenant on the battlefield. I'm an ex-Marine, therefore I cannot know defeat! I will win; Johnny will be dead. No more lost memory; no more shameful behavior; no more violent outbursts; no more longing for simple peace.*"

9 P.M.: *"Ann is being very brave and helpful. She believes in my complete cure. She said Dr. Allison is convinced also. I sure hope so.*

"I can't put up with this much longer. Johnny is winning and I can't let that happen. This has to be my final battle. I shall win! Johnny has won almost every skirmish and battle since the beginning. He destroys every accomplishment of mine. He has brought me shame and dishonor. He has kept my poor wife in a state of confusion. Every time I'm a winner, he makes me into a loser. My physical, mental, and moral deterioration has been his single goal. He haunts me most of the time. He whispers to me sometimes so softly that I confuse it with my own thoughts. Sometimes I can't separate good from evil or right from wrong. All I know is that for Johnny to live, I must die."

Monday, April 26. 9:00 A.M.: *"I feel a little depressed this morning. I seem to have doubts about my cure. I wonder if it really can be. It seems that all my life, failure immediately follows success. It overshadows and destroys that success. Yet I keep picking up the pieces and trying again. Hundreds of times I've picked up the pieces and tried again.*

"I'm tired now but I must push on. The week or two that I stay in this hospital could be the turning point of my life.

"Johnny, I know you can read this. You have had your last stand. You're through! Your death will be my rebirth!

"As I sit here I figure I am as sane as the sanest. Yet I know I would break down and change very soon after being on the outside. Almost all my life I have wanted to commit myself. I have always known something was wrong with me, but I would rationalize myself out of it. I was probably afraid I might have to face the truth. Yet I don't know what that truth is.

"Is it a fear of the unknown? If I'm so normal, how come I've had so many jobs? I listed all the jobs I have had and the total came to 31. Then I listed all the different houses in which I've lived and it came to 29.

"Even the simple pleasures in life have escaped me because of that God-damned Johnny! I poured thousands and

thousands of dollars into attorney fees and fines. I continue to pay expensive doctor fees just because of the S.O.B. Johnny. He says he is going to ruin me. He says he is going to break me until I have no will of my own. He's almost won but not quite. Either he dies in the next two weeks or we both die! If I kill myself—destroy my body—he dies too!

"The world will be better off. Ann and the kids will be rid of their problem and my employer's life insurance will pay all my bills while leaving a good nest egg for Ann.

"I'll have to make it look like an accident. With my driving record that wouldn't be hard to do. It would be quite believable.

"It's stupid for me to talk like this. I'm not going to commit suicide! I'm going to win this battle and go home a single, whole person with full command of my own destiny.

"As I think back over the years it's hard for me to remember even one moment of happiness. The closest to joy I have experienced was watching the birth and success of my kids. Each one is developing into a good person. The future belongs to them and is in good hands.

"Most of my memories are of my father drilling the idea into my head that the end justified the means. I remember his successes and failures; his inability to get close to me. How I longed to know him . . .

"And my mother's death. Her death ended her misery. It was so senseless. Four others died in that accident. Three college girls with their whole life in front of them and her boyfriend I never got to know.

"Then there was the funeral and the family meeting. Greed, everywhere greed. She had so little, yet they fought over who would get what dress and who would get what bill.

"Everyone said I was cold at the funeral. They said I had no feelings because I didn't cry. I don't remember much about the funeral except what I was told. I suspect that cool, efficient personality everyone mentioned was Phil. He seems to take control during times of stress.

"I could never be what my father wanted. He wanted a partner in his quest for notoriety. He wanted me to be able

to go out night after night and talk his language. He wanted me to enjoy the same things he did, but it just wasn't in me. I tried, but I couldn't measure up to his standards. Even my mother's death was ultimately my father's fault, yet he couldn't prevent it either. She couldn't withstand his pressure on her. It is said that each man kills the thing he loves. Maybe that's the way it was with them."

April 27. 10:30 A.M.: *"Depressed again this morning. I try and think about my problem but my mind refuses to work. It's as though it doesn't want to deal with my reality.*

"I have so many things going for me that it's almost a crime for me to be depressed or feel sorry for myself. I have a good wife, three healthy children, a nice house in the country, good physical health, reasonable looks, above-average intelligence, profitable skills in selling and management. What more could anyone want?

"Yet I have a constant dread of failure. Johnny seems to gnaw at me constantly. I always feel as if doom is just around the corner. Using hindsight, I now realize that Johnny has been trying to come out for several weeks. He wasn't satisfied with just being out long enough to get me jailed on a drunk-driving charge. I know Johnny's just waiting for the opportunity to take full charge."

3 P.M.: *"Dr. Allison called me for an age-regression session. We covered ages 16 and 17. I felt rather wrung out when it was over. The doctor said that most of my normal emotions were suppressed and that I should try harder to recognize them for what they are.*

"A woman just walked by with her husband comforting her while she cried. How I wish I could cry like that! I wish I could let it all hang out!"

4 P.M.: *"I showered, shaved, and changed clothes. Sitting here feeling refreshed and observing the trees swaying gently in the Spring breeze I ask myself what the hell I'm doing here. There's nothing wrong with me. All I have to do is to keep going on just like I am.*

"How soon I'm forgetting that I turned myself in to this place. I'm trying to forget the depression that almost immo-

bilized me. I'm avoiding facing the hundreds and thousands of times I said everything was fine; that I had no more problems, only to discover my world had once again become a nightmare.

"Sometimes I feel like I belong to another time and place, maybe even another world.

Sometimes I want to talk to a redwood tree and ask it to give me some of its wisdom; the wisdom that allows it to stand through centuries of turmoil and strife while still remaining straight and proud. I think of the great and giant battles it has fought just to keep a piece of the sky. I see it slowly healing wounds from forest fires long past. It has fought starvation during droughts and survived, only to have a harsh wind bend it almost to the point of breaking. Then it snaps back straighter and stronger than before. When I hear someone say 'It's only a tree,' I realize how ignorant man can be.

"Am I an evil person who should be cut off from mankind and destroyed in the Hell-Fire of Biblical description? Yet how can I be all evil and still love the sweetness of Spring, the colors of the petals of a pansy, the giant redwood trees? How can I be a father and a husband? Or should all that be destroyed too? All of these are parts of my personality.

"A woman patient just came into the area where I'm writing. She is playing simple melodies on a guitar. My mind drifts off to another place where the evening is cool and fires emit a soft orange light reflecting from kind faces singing a song of peace.

"I'm feeling tired, depressed. Maybe I should lie down for a while."

The next entry was in a different handwriting. Dana had no memory of how it had gotten into the journal. It was a message from Johnny:

"I just read what you wrote, you stupid son-of-a-bitch! Reality is hate! The more you hate, the more you win. I hate you so I'll win. I'm going to take a look down the hospital and see what a soft life you have. Don't worry, Buddy, I'm going to screw things up for you. Oops, here come the nurses. Goodbye." It was signed *"Johnny."*

Dana continued making entries:

"Now I'm writing notes to myself. Why can't Johnny just go away? This whole thing is crazy. I guess that's why I'm in the crazy ward."

April 28: *"This afternoon the dance therapist came again. This time we played drawing circles and symbols in the air with sticks. After about 30 minutes of light exercises we ended the session. If anybody on the outside saw me doing this, they would understand why I was here."*

April 29: *"The first thing I was thinking about this morning was a plan for getting out of here. The only two stumbling blocks in my fantasy are the lack of money and lack of a car. The door isn't locked since everyone is here voluntarily.*

"The more I thought about my escape plan, the more I recognized it was Johnny thinking. I had better not get caught up in it. If I left here Johnny would take over at the first opportunity. That would negate all the days I've been here and I'd be breaking another promise I had made to myself—the promise that only one of us would be leaving here. There can be no truce and no compromise, only victory.

"There are times when I'm not certain why I'm here. It's so easy for me to forget the past. It's so easy for me to fake optimism. Too many years as a salesman, I guess. I can be cheerful when I'm sad, like the image of a clown.

"Sometimes I wonder if I, Dana, am the real self—the real personality. It's a new thought and it bothers me. I wonder if buried real deep inside my mind is another personality—the one I was born with. Is such a personality the reason I have this longing for something different? Is this a truth I have yet to face?

"It's a frightening thought. If there is another personality, then I am doomed just like Peter and Phil.

"And if this other me surfaces, will he remember my life? Will he remember my wife and kids and love them as I do? And if he does exist, then are my wife and kids also his wife and kids or must he start life as a totally different person? Maybe the fact that I've been so tired lately is a sign that my

days are numbered just like the others. If this is so, will the first me emerge as an undeveloped immature child or has he been developing and maturing in silence in some protected recess of my mind?

"I wonder if the emergence of the first me would mean my death. Or will I be like an individual drop of water that loses its identity when it hits the pond, but survives as an addition to the whole."

3:30 P.M.: *"The doctor said my thoughts about a hidden me are possible. Most of the therapy session today we just talked about theories. He left my head full of thoughts, some of them strange. But this is a strange state of being.*

"One of the things he suggested was that the original me was laying back in my mind, unable to make a judgment between Johnny and Dana. If he comes out and takes my qualities to mix with his own, then I live on in a way. But if he comes out and adopts Johnny's bad qualities, then Johnny lives on.

"The doctor feels that if there really is another personality—the original me—and he comes out while Johnny still exists, he might not be able to overcome the evil. I've had so many years of living with him that I'm the only person who can defeat him.

"This whole line of philosophical thinking scares me a bit. It's an interesting theory—good versus evil. But I'm not certain I'm ready to find out whether or not I will be able to continue my existence."

CHAPTER 23

Dana was sitting on the patio just off one wing of the Crisis Intervention Ward. It was three stories above the ground and surrounded by a high wall to prevent would-be suicides from trying to take their own lives. However, breaks in the wall enabled Dana to look out over the hospital grounds. He was writing his observations when he lost consciousness for a moment. When he was again in control, Jerry had written:

"You have part of the truth. I cannot give you the whole truth. I cannot give you anything. You can only talk to Henry and his time is not yet. You have been good to him and I have a place for you when the time comes. I now choose to give you another piece of truth. You will sit at my side with Phil and Peter, guiding the affairs of Henry. No man on earth will have a better team to guide him to his destination in this life. But first Henry must choose between good and evil. He must choose between Johnny and us. This must be an act of free will. He does not know of this message, nor will he until the choice is made. This is the first and last time I will speak until the battle is over."

The words shocked Dana. He knew about Jerry from the doctor's therapy. He was apparently the personality created to unite the others and help them become a whole person.

If the words were true, the implication was that Dana's thoughts about an original personality—Henry—were true. And the mention of the unity of Peter, Phil, Dana, and Jerry tended to confirm the idea of the personalities merging like drops of water forming a puddle. Yet everything seemed so strange to him. And if there was a Henry and the message was wrong, Dana knew he might die.

After reading and thinking about the message for a moment, Dana again blacked out. When he awakened, the writing in front of him was Johnny's. It said:

"You son-of-a-bitch! The war is on. Look about you and see how often I have won! No power within you can beat me. Remember that there is no Henry or Jerry—just you and me. And when that battle is over, I will be left. Goodbye, you bastard."

April 30: *"I woke up this morning denying the thoughts of yesterday. They were the stupid fantasies of a sick mind.*

"I saw the doctor after breakfast and we discussed the theory a little more. Then he age-regressed me to 21 and I relived my pending marriage to Ann and the other experiences of the period.

"A new thought just crossed my mind. When I came to the hospital I was like an expectant mother. I'm going to give birth to a new me—my own baby. I wish to God I knew what it would be.

"Johnny, let's talk. You and me go back a long way together. We've been battling for supremacy of this body for years. But as long as I'm around, you're not going to win. I'm tired but I believe you're even more tired. I think that is why you are putting up such a tough last stand. Why don't you and me call a truce after all these years? Why don't we let Henry choose between us? If he chooses me, I will merge with him and he can be reborn. If he chooses you, then you

merge with him and he can be reborn. The last rule we must play by is simply this: whoever is not chosen must leave the scene and go wherever non-persons go. There's no certainty who will win. It is a gamble, though with as many trips to Las Vegas as you've taken, you certainly like to gamble."

This was followed by a message from Johnny. It read:
"Fuck you, you son of a bitch!"

Dana wrote: *"Come on, Johnny, let's bring this thing to a head and may the best man win. If you think you are the best man, then you know that you will win. How about it?"*

Johnny wrote: *"I'm thinkin'."*

"Okay. Take your time," wrote Dana.

The last note from Johnny read simply, *"Goodbye for now."*

Dana finished the morning entries with: *"I guess I'll have to give him some time to think. I hope he is not playing another trick on me and making it easier for him to come out. That's a worrisome question. I've asked him to gamble so I guess I'll have to gamble, too."*

4:30 P.M.: *"The dance therapist girl has come and gone. The exercises relaxed me so much I was a little afraid that I might doze off and Johnny would take control. Fortunately it didn't happen.*

"Kate is in here with her guitar again. She's playing a last song before she leaves the ward. I hope that she finds on the outside whatever she is looking for. I hope that all the patients eventually find what they are looking for. They're all lost souls at a way station, trying to find their way somewhere.

"It's funny, but I think I know where I'm going. I'm going to the Yellow Room, the inner chamber, the sanctum of the soul. I now believe that I will keep my identity. Another step up the ladder that eventually turns back on itself.

"Is the peace I am beginning to feel a preparation for my departure? Am I assuming victory over Johnny? I can't assume this. The choice must still be made. I guess all I can do is wait for Johnny's decision and Henry's choice. I must leave it at that.

"The time for decision is growing near."

Saturday, May 1. 10:00 A.M.: *"I have been here a week today. No question that there has been plenty of progress with my case. I found out that Henry and Dana are separate personalities. I'm Dana and my purpose for being is about to cease. When my purpose ceases, I must disappear and Henry will be reborn after 40 years.*

"The doctor was here the first thing this morning and our sessions started at 8 A.M. More age regression, this time to 22 and 23. More Johnny incidents and Phil used automatic writing to say that Johnny's outbursts were designed to destroy my successes. It's like a private war between Johnny and me. Phil's main job is to protect the body. He seems to come out when the body is threatened."

Dana continued writing, discussing his thoughts and his dreams, when he suddenly became depressed and lost consciousness for a moment. When he awakened he found a note reading: *"I accept and I'll win this war because I offer more excitement and fun. You offer nothing. Goodbye. Johnny."*

The note surprised Dana. He wrote: *"Thanks, Johnny. The contest begins."*

Dana continued in his journal: *"I know now why it has been hard for me to get close to people. I'd fear they would see that I am not a complete person. They would know how superficial I really am.*

"I've been writing these pages as a means of searching for the truth about myself. Now I believe that there is a second purpose that is just as important. That purpose is to leave Henry a record of what transpired to bring him forth into the world again.

"All my years of turmoil and strife, all the battles have had the single purpose of bringing forth one whole human being. How important must Henry be to have all this struggle go on for him? I doubt that he will ever appreciate it.

"I've likened this hospital ward to a way station for lost souls, but it also has the quality of a cocoon. We enter here as worms and emerge as butterflies. It's also a battlefield of good and evil. This place is many things to many people.

"For me it has been all three, for it is here that I found the

truth. How painful the truth is, yet it is ultimately good. I crawled here and Henry will emerge. But first there will be the great battle between the evil forces possessing his body and the good forces who are also in control. I just hope that the time-worn concept of good triumphing over evil has a basis in fact."

5:00 P.M.: *"Ann just left and though I wanted to see her as often as possible, I have run out of things to say. I know she is disturbed because I don't give her honest progress reports. But how can I? What'll I say? The man you married is about to pass on to oblivion leaving only an essence behind. How can I expect her to understand? It even boggles my mind and I am living the experience. But I have underestimated her many times before and maybe she can adjust to yet another shock. I hope Henry can give her the deep love and understanding that I have been incapable of all these years. God knows that she deserves the best. I hope Henry can do what I was not able to do. I will tell Henry that I have done a good job with Linda and Mark. Scott, so brave and courageous, I leave to Henry to finish raising. It is a responsibility Henry must accept or I will find some way to haunt him.*

"I guess my threats against Henry are meaningless. Besides, we all share the same heart. If he looks inside himself, he'll find my dedication to the children.

"I guess the way my writing is going now, I'm beginning to sound like I'm writing my last will and testament. Shall I start by saying, 'Being of sound mind, I give to Henry all my possessions, the best of Phil, Peter, and myself, and this notebook?

"To Ann, Linda, Mark, and Scott I give Henry. To Dr. Allison I give thanks for the destruction of Johnny, though I had to be sacrificed in the process. I also give to Dr. Allison the encouragement to practice his kind of medicine no matter what. I believe I have nothing else to give. May 1, 1976. Signed, Dana Hawksworth.

"My time is near. I want to last through Sunday night so Ann can have the benefit of Dr. Allison's consoling."

Sunday, May 2, 1976. 10:00 A.M.: *"Last night was a bad*

night. My mind kept wondering about the shock that Ann will suffer when Dr. Allison talks to her. Before she left last night I tried to prepare her by referring to 'the man who walks out of here.' I felt she had absorbed this, at least on the emotional level. But I empathized with how her mind must be experiencing all sorts of wild and bizarre thoughts after I told her that I am not a real person but rather an alter-personality of Henry's. I was created to serve as Johnny's opponent in the 40-year battle that has been raging 24 hours a day and is only now coming to an end.

"I don't think that Johnny realizes that even if he wins he will lose. No matter which one of us Henry chooses to be like, we both lose. If he goes with Johnny, I will cease to exist on a conscious level and Johnny will become a major part of Henry. Henry will be the only possessor of the body.

"Another new thought crossed my mind. Perhaps the reason my emotional range is so limited is because when I experience any extremes of emotion, Johnny can take control. Perhaps I have deliberately narrowed my own emotional range during the last 40 years so no one else would take charge of the body. Perhaps I have been afraid to be as tender and loving towards Ann as I have seen other men be towards their wives because I felt that trying to express tenderness would just bring Peter out. And if Peter was in control, his weakness would enable Johnny to push him aside and take over. Perhaps this is an answer to my behavior over the years. Perhaps the hospital therapy is helping me bring forth knowledge that has been buried within me."

May 3. 11:00 A.M.: *"This morning Johnny came out and had breakfast. I barely remember eating at all. Another patient said I looked awfully mean. I took over right after breakfast and Johnny came out again at the community meeting where the patients and the staff discuss their mutual problems. He retreated quickly, though. I wish I knew what's on his mind. I don't believe Johnny can stay out long without booze. But the fact that he came out at all and that I feel so tired is something new."*

2 P.M.: *"I didn't know the end was going to be so painful. It's too late, no turning back, I'm committed. It is the winter*

of my discontent. Spring is near. Time of rebirth. Please Henry, come. I don't want to suffer any more. What's happening? I know I have to suffer more before it's time. It's not time yet."

At four o'clock that day a nurse found Dana on the patio experiencing what appeared to be an epileptic fit, though it was not caused by epilepsy. His fingernails had dug into his arms until they had punctured the skin and caused it to bleed. When the nurse grabbed his shoulders he lost consciousness, then came out of the seizure. He awakened feeling completely disoriented and had to be helped to his room. There Jerry took control and asked the nurse for a pencil and piece of paper. On it he wrote: "Dana has been to Hell. Johnny and the evil entity he represented have been consumed and damned. Dana has emerged clean and ready to bring Henry forth."

The words made little sense to Dana and I still don't fully understand them. However, from that moment on Johnny would never again control my body. He had gone forever. I was left with the ability to express a normal amount of anger instead of being totally consumed by hate as Johnny had been.

Dr. Allison arrived a short time later and went to Dana's room. He had him lie down on the bed and put him under hypnosis. He told him to go to sleep and find Henry. Dana said he would, then told the doctor "goodbye."

"Henry Hawksworth, wake up," said the doctor in a gentle but firm voice.

The child/man on the bed moved slightly. He had been having a dream about his birthday party and his Charlie McCarthy doll. Johnny, in the dream, had told him he had smashed Charlie's face and buried him in the backyard because he was dead. The child had been scared by the words. He wished Peter Pan would come and take him to Never-Never Land where Johnny wouldn't be able to bother him.

"Henry Hawksworth, open your eyes."

The child/man on the bed did as he was told. The light bothered him, though, and he had to shield his face to keep his eyes from hurting. He could make out a doctor in the room. He wondered if he was sick.

The child/man looked about him. There were two chairs, a desk, a small table, and a bed—all of them strange. He wasn't in his own room. The furniture was strange to him.

The nurse dimmed the light. "Henry, is that better?" asked the doctor.

"Yes," said the child/man. His voice was loud and deep, like his father's. It startled the child/man. It wasn't the voice he remembered having when he laid down to take his nap. But it was his voice—my voice—the voice of Henry Hawksworth, who was being reborn at three years of age in a forty-three-year-old body.

"Where's my mommy and daddy?" I asked.

"They're not here," said the doctor.

"They're dead?" I was astonished to hear myself say such words.

"Yes," said the doctor. "What's the last thing you remember, Henry?"

"My Charlie McCarthy doll. It wasn't in my toy box, but before I could look for it, I had to take my nap."

"You've been asleep a long time." The doctor placed a chair next to the bed and sat on it.

"Do you know the story of Rip Van Winkle?" asked the doctor.

A picture of an old man with a long white beard flashed into my mind. I knew no one had told me the story before I went to sleep, yet somehow I understood what the doctor was talking about. "Yes, I know it."

"You are something like Rip Van Winkle. You've slept a long time."

I was puzzled for a moment, then I touched my face. I was relieved to discover I had no beard. Then I noticed my feet. They were big and seemed very far away.

I looked at my hand, then compared it with the doctor's. My hand was so big! I had to study it for a minute. It had never been so big before.

"My mother and father are dead and I've been asleep a long time."

"Yes, Henry, you've been asleep forty years."

I thought of Rip Van Winkle again. Then images of the hospital, the doctor, and the nurses came to my mind. It was like remembering a dream.

"Welcome back, Henry."

"Thank you," I said, automatically.

The doctor picked up Dana's notebook on the small bedside table. "This book was left to you by someone to help understand what has happened." The doctor selected his words carefully. I had the body and the vocabulary of a forty-three-year-old man but the understanding of a three-year-old child.

I was awed by the book as he put it back on the table. Then he asked, "Do you remember anything about Dana?"

The name jarred me. My mind was blank for a minute. Then I remembered that Dana was my middle name. It seemed a silly question for the doctor to ask.

"Don't read the book until the nurse or I say it's all right."

"Yes." I didn't think I knew how to read.

The doctor had to leave. I was frightened by his going because he represented security to me. But the nurse was friendly and she took me around to the different rooms.

It was odd. Things I had never seen before were somehow familiar. The box with the moving picture screen was a television set. The bathroom and shower all were familiar, though I didn't know when I had seen them before. Even some of the other patients seemed to know me and I them.

It was all so strange. Memories were flooding my mind; memories of things I had never known yet, which were a part of my life.

On May 5, I met Ann, the woman with whom my personalities had been living for more than twenty years. I knew her the moment I saw her and she was even more beautiful than the memories I had inherited. I felt a rush of emotion of an intensity Dana had never been able to experience. It was love; the first love for another human being I had ever felt as a complete individual. The feeling seemed to overwhelm my entire being.

On Ann's next visit she brought my son Scott with her. I was scared about meeting him. I had rehearsed all the things I would say when I first saw him. I was going to be the calm, cool, level-headed parent, even though I was still part child myself.

I didn't say a thing I had rehearsed except, "How was school?" The rest just flowed. I couldn't stop looking at Scott. I had a new feeling when I saw him, a little like what I felt when I first saw Ann, except that it was different. My mind told me it was the kind of love a father feels for his son. I knew I'd feel the same kind of love when I met Mark.

I didn't know what I'd feel when I met Linda. Perhaps the special feeling a father has for his daughter was different from what he experiences with his sons. It was all so strange and yet so wonderful.

The next few days passed quickly. I was allowed to leave the hospital for increasing periods of time. Ann took me home for meals and I explored the house and the neighborhood in which I lived. Everything I saw and touched triggered memories of the past—some good, some rather unpleasant. Yet everything was new. I knew what had happened, where I lived, and what I owned when Dana was in control, but I, Henry, had never really seen any of it.

Ann brought out the family picture album and I got to study twenty years of experiences I had never really had. I saw my life, yet it was someone else's life. I tried to absorb everything I could until my mind became exhausted and I could think no more. Then I fell asleep, letting all the memories and experiences find their proper place and leave me ready for new experiences the next day.

By Tuesday, May 11, I was permanently living at home. Linda had returned from college and seeing her was a wonderful emotional experience. As I suspected, my feelings for her, my daughter, were different from my feelings for the others but equally intense.

Linda had promised to teach me to drive a car. I was quite nervous behind the wheel and pleased with her patience. It was a strange feeling to know that Dana had taught her to drive and suddenly she was teaching me. Not many daughters get that chance.

That Friday I did some housework. It took me three hours to repair a broken screen door and I perspired enough while doing it to fill a swimming pool. Ann commented that Dana had almost never perspired, even when working harder than I did and in hotter weather. Apparently my body chemistry had changed somewhat in the fusion.

My relationship with Ann intensified almost at once. She had been as close to a complete breakdown as Dana when he had entered the hospital, though he hadn't known it. For her the change had been miraculous and rejuvenating. She was relaxed; no longer fearful. We were like young lovers those first days, experiencing an intense type of passion normally felt only by newlyweds. Our relationship has been reborn.

The following Wednesday I had an appointment with the personnel manager of the department store where I had worked as Dana. I was frightened by what might happen since Johnny had caused such trouble.

The personnel manager said that he did not fully understand my illness. Everyone in the department, however, as well as the store manager and the Los Angeles branch manager of the chain, all had spoken on my behalf. He said that so long as I was cured, my job was waiting for me.

It was hard for me to comprehend his words. Even after the destructive violence of Johnny everyone was willing to give me the chance to continue. I didn't know how to thank them or repay them for their kindness. I was overwhelmed, yet joyous and determined to prove their faith was well founded.

Then on Thursday, May 20, the last traces of my alter-personalities were destroyed. I awakened shortly before seven and heard Scott say he saw smoke coming from the new floor heater we had just installed.

When I checked the heater I, too, thought I detected smoke coming through the frame. Rather than take any chances, I turned off the heater and had Scott bring me a glass of water. Some of the wood was glowing and I doused it immediately. Closer inspection, however, revealed flames still inside the walls. I had Scott call the fire department.

We saw Ann and the rest of the family safely out of the house, then Scott and I rounded up the family pets. We gathered the two cats, the dogs, and the bird, rushing them outside where they would be safe. Then I grabbed the garden hose and took it through the front door, trying to spray the wall that had burst into flames. It was no use. In a few minutes flames were shooting through every part of the house.

The fire department arrived quickly and the blaze was out in less than thirty minutes, but the house was in ruins. The possessions of Dana, Peter, Phil, and Johnny had been destroyed. My past was burned away. The foundation that remained was, in a sense, the foundation for my new life. Only those things that mattered—my family and the pets —had been saved.

CHAPTER **24**

It was the middle of June when I had to answer for the last of Johnny's actions. The drunk-driving charge he had received during the final days of his existence was being taken to court. My attorney and I had decided to fight it, an unusual approach for so seemingly simple a case. There might one day be other court cases involving former mental patients who had been cured of multiple personality problems, and we felt if we showed that the actions had been Johnny's and Johnny no longer existed, there would be no case.

The initial testimony was from the principals involved —the arresting officer and the technicians who tried to administer the tests. Then Dr. Allison was called to the stand and asked to list his credentials. When he had clearly established his expertise, the most important portion of the trial began.

"Do you have any special interests in the field of psychiatry?" the defense attorney asked Dr. Allison.

"The multiple personality phenomenon," said the doctor.

"Are you considered a specialist on the subject?"

"I am doing a book on the subject and am considered one of the authorities in California."

Dr. Allison then explained that I had been a patient of his since March of 1975 when I had come to see him about receiving Lithium treatments for a manic-depressive condition. I had seen other psychiatrists before him, he said, and twice been diagnosed as manic-depressive. He had started me on the Lithium treatment but found that my behavior problems were only slightly modified.

After a couple of months of unsatisfactory treatment, he went on, he had used hypnosis to probe my subconscious. He explained that the first sessions were not successful but that the fourth time it was tried, Dana blurted out: "I don't drink, Johnny does." It was at that session that the true story of my mind began to unfold.

Then the question of Johnny arose, and the doctor explained that Johnny's sole purpose in life had been to try to destroy Dana. He had wanted to break down Dana's personality until it was too weak to resist any longer. The doctor stressed that Johnny had been driving the car the night of the drunk-driving arrest. He had bragged about it, in fact, during a therapy session following the incident.

"Is it possible for you to demonstrate the multiple personalities?" asked my attorney.

"I can use age regression to take Henry back to the time when they were in existence," said the doctor. "I can take him to a period before the fusion and call out the personalities of Peter and Phil."

"Would you demonstrate for the court?"

"I object, Your Honor," said the District Attorney. "The demonstration will serve no purpose unless he brings out this Johnny he alleges was operating the car at the time of the arrest."

The judge was curious, however. He said to proceed with the demonstration. The objection was overruled.

Dr. Allison placed two chairs so that they were facing each other. He took one and asked me to sit on the other.

Then he used hypnosis to age-regress me to a period before fusion had taken place. He called out Peter.

The people in the courtroom were startled by the change in me. My eyes widened and Peter drew his feet up so he was squatting on the chair. Then he tried to lean back as though he thought the chair would allow him to rock. (One of the chairs in the doctor's office reclined and could be made to rock slightly by leaning back, then sitting forward, then leaning back again.) Peter was disappointed in the chair. He asked the doctor if it was broken, indicating he thought he was in the doctor's office.

"No, Peter, it's not broken. This is a slightly different chair than usual and I'm afraid you won't be able to rock."

Peter began wriggling. He looked down at his feet and asked the doctor why Dana hadn't worn his shoes with the shiny buckles. He was referring to a pair of loafers frequently worn during visits to the psychiatrist's office.

"What are you doing these days, Peter?" asked Dr. Allison.

"Not much. I'm kind of scared. Something's going to happen soon that scares me." (He was referring to the fusion.)

"What would you like to be doing right now?" asked the doctor.

"I think I'd like to climb a tree and try to guess what it's thinking about. But don't worry, I'd climb it real carefully so I wouldn't hurt even the tiniest branch. Trees are nice. It wouldn't be fun to climb them if I thought they might feel bad."

"Peter, tell me what you think of Johnny."

Peter's face grew serious. "I'm scared of Johnny. I'm real scared of Johnny. He's bad."

"How bad is Johnny?"

Peter's expression remained serious. He took his arms and spread them apart as far as they would go. "That bad!"

There were a few more questions and then Phil was brought out. He was relaxed, mature, and serious. When the doctor asked him the date, he said it was Wednesday, October 2, 1975.

Dr. Allison then questioned Phil about Johnny.

"That son-of-a-bitch has given me nothing but hell over the years!" said Phil. "He keeps getting into one damn-fool mess after another and I have to rescue him before we're all killed. The bastard's evil—pure evil. I'll be glad when you get rid of him, Doc, though I'm going to be saddened by the fact that I won't have a chance at living without him. You'll be making all of us one person and I'd kind of like to be by myself for a while without Johnny being around."

The doctor asked a few more questions, then brought me out of hypnosis. The demonstration was over. I returned to my seat and the doctor was questioned by the District Attorney.

The questioning was extensive. The D. A. wanted to prove that some sort of trick had been used.

"Isn't it true, Dr. Allison, that the testimony you have given about the defendant came directly from him and you have no other person to collaborate it?" asked the D. A.

"Yes, that is essentially true, except for what his wife and children have told me."

"Then the diagnosis you made for the defendant is based only on what the defendant, himself, told you!"

"Yes, that is the way psychiatry works. It's a patient-and-doctor relationship."

"In other words, your diagnosis could be just what the defendant wanted you to believe."

The doctor thought a moment, then said, "I guess that is possible, but I doubt it very much. It is part of the psychiatric training to detect what is true and what is false. Besides, a patient will seldom spend $50 a week just to fulfill the challenge of fooling the doctor over a period of a year or more."

"But it is possible?"

"Yes, anything is possible. But it is my professional opinion that Henry Hawksworth was a bona fide classical case of hysterical disassociation or multiple personality and is now cured."

The District Attorney questioned the doctor about the cure, then decided to change his tactics. "What did you mean when you said Johnny and these other alter-egos are unconscious?" he asked. "You alleged Johnny was driving the car and I saw the other personalities behaving like normal people here in the courtroom. Phil and Peter didn't look unconscious to me."

"Both consciousness and unconsciousness can be many things," said Dr. Allison. "Unconsciousness means not being conscious. Unlike law, which has limited itself to just a single definition for each state, medicine talks about many altered states of consciousness.

"Let me put it this way—if Henry's body was an automobile, then the day of the arrest Johnny took Dana out of the driver's seat and locked him in the trunk so he wouldn't know what was going on. Then Johnny got behind the wheel. You might say the incident was like a change of drivers."

"No matter what he calls himself," said the D.A., his voice rising in anger and frustration, "a person identified as Dana was driving the car in a state of physical mobility and therefore was conscious. Isn't that right?"

"Would you call a sleeping person unconscious?" asked Dr. Allison.

"Certainly. But answer my question."

"Then talking in one's sleep or sleepwalking is an unconscious mobilization of the body."

"Doctor, are you saying that Dana was not drunk, regardless of what name he was using? Are you saying that the alcohol was only affecting his body?"

"To repeat myself, I'm saying that Dana was unconscious or in an altered state of consciousness. It was Johnny who did the drinking and I'm not sure that Johnny was drunk."

"What do you mean? You heard the testimony of the police officer on the case. How can you deny that he was drunk? Are you some kind of expert on drunkenness too? You heard the testimony that Dana couldn't tell the officer even what time it was, and that is one of the standard tests."

"I've worked a lot with alcoholics and have testified as an expert witness for both the state and the defense several times on matters of alcoholic conduct," said the doctor calmly. "Yes, I heard the tape made during the arrest and I felt that Johnny's answers were crisp, well thought out, and obviously designed to bait the officer. I heard no indication of slurred speech or any of the hesitations typical of a drunk person. In regard to the time problem, it was night and dark. Both vehicles had their lights on and yet Johnny said it was twelve noon. If you are sober enough to answer the question, you are sober enough to know the difference between night and day. I believe that again he was just baiting the officer."

The District Attorney was determined to convict me. He knew he had to discredit my doctor.

"Dr. Allison, how do you know it was dark? I suppose you remember last March and the time it got dark then? I suppose you are an expert at this, also?"

"I don't have to be an expert. I'm just taking the word of your own witness."

"If Dana, I mean Henry . . . Or is it Johnny, Phil, or Peter . . . Who in the hell is on trial here?"

"I believe it is the man sitting at the table—Mr. Hawksworth."

The District Attorney was becoming increasingly frustrated. He couldn't discredit the doctor so he decided to try to discredit the concept of multiple personality. Finally, after several minutes of this, Dr. Allison said, "We're just going around in circles. I have answered your questions as precisely as possible. It seems obvious that we are having a problem with words."

The questioning continued a few more minutes, then the judge decided to end the trial for the day. He asked if there were any more witnesses to be introduced or if the attorneys wished to make any closing arguments. They didn't.

The judge proceeded to read his decision, a decision he had started writing even before the D. A.'s final questions had been asked. He had been convinced by the demonstration of age regression and the testimony of Dr. Allison. He said that it is the intent of the law to protect society from the drunken driver. The law was not concerned with alter-personalities but with whole people. From the testimony presented, he was fairly certain that Henry Hawksworth had not been drunk at the time the arrest was made. Henry Hawksworth, therefore, was declared "Not Guilty!"

And what of the future? It hardly seems to matter. Because of the love of my family, the compassion of my employer, and the skills of my psychiatrist, I shall face it as a whole man. It may be bitter or it may bring continued happiness and joy, but either way I will experience it fully and that will make it worthwhile.

The nightmare of my forty-year "nap" is over.

Appendix

Introduction

Mrs. Donna Reed, CGA, is a certified handwriting analyst who lives in Tucson, Arizona. She has studied handwriting analysis under the guidance of Tucson instructor Beryl Hamilton as well as with the International Graphoanalysis Society, Chicago, Illinois, from which she received certification as a professional handwriting analyst.

Mrs. Reed teaches classes in handwriting analysis, is a lecturer, does personal analyses, and has been employed by a national personnel firm.

Mr. Ted Schwarz gave Mrs. Reed xerox copies of the handwriting of Peter, Jerry, Johnny, and Dana. After the initial work was done, she was given an original current specimen of the patient's handwriting, which was incorporated into the final analysis and comparison.

Each of the four hands was analyzed separately and a brief personality sketch written. Comparisons of the five (patient's current original included) were then done.

The amount of writing available for analysis: twelve lines from Peter, seven lines from Jerry, seven lines from Johnny, seven lines from Dana, and twelve lines from Henry. Only parts of the available handwriting are reproduced here.

EMOTIONAL STRUCTURE

As Shown On Perspectrographs

PETER

Withdrawn	Objective	Moderately Responsive	Very Responsive
6%	37%	53%	4%
FA	AB	BC	CD

JERRY

Objective	Moderately Responsive	Very Responsive	Impulsive
12%	22%	50%	16%
AB	BC	CD	DE

JOHNNY

Withdrawn	Objective	Moderately Responsive	Very Responsive	Impulsive	Very Impulsive
4%	24%	43%	17%	10%	2%
FA	AB	BC	CD	DE	E+

DANA

Withdrawn	Objective	Moderately Responsive	Very Responsive	Impulsive
5%	25%	49%	16%	5%
FA	AB	BC	CD	DE

HENRY

Objective	Moderately Responsive	Very Responsive	Impulsive
8%	24%	56%	12%
AB	BC	CD	DE

Analysis of Individual Hands

Peter—Age 7

Peter's handwriting shows him to be a very precocious young boy. In fact, the handwriting factors indicate that Peter has a mental and emotional age closer to that of an eleven- to thirteen-year-old.

On a
Forest Morning
as the golden sunbeams of the brand-new day
reincarnate the sleeping, forest hues,
the hush is broken by the cawing Jay
Raccoons have made their pre-dawn rendezvous
in bedrooms on creeksides and riverbanks)
while the Quail start with their ʔ.T... cries

Emotional Structure. Perspectrograph # 1 reveals Peter's emotional structure to be 6% withdrawn (FA), 37% objective (AB), 53% moderately responsive (BC), and 4% very responsive (CD). Basically, Peter is an objective person who prefers to make decisions based on logic rather than feeling.

Thinking Patterns. Peter is a logical thinker, preferring to think in sequence. He likes things to "make sense" and best understands concepts that build on previous steps. At the same time, there is a lot of creativity in Peter's thinking structure. He likes to take existing situations, rearrange them, change, add to, take from, etc., and create a new and different final product. Peter would not be considered a quick learner but is one who learns thoroughly and thinks in creative ways. One aspect of his creativity is shown in his ability to use his hands well.

Personality Profile. Peter's creative ability (with his mind as well as his hands) is one of his strongest characteristics. He also pays close attention to details and is loyal to what he believes to be right. He is quite independent in his thinking (rather unusual in a child so young) and shows some organizational ability. He is idealistic in his goal-setting and has the necessary willpower to reach his goals. He feels quite possessive about what is his, which includes responsibilities, people, and things.

Peter has a tendency to talk a great deal, which could be a positive or a negative force in his personality, depending on how he uses this trait.

There is a small amount of temper exhibited as well as some degree of stubbornness.

A deliberate attempt at self-control is shown. Peter is also sensitive to the criticism of people. He tends to be generous to others as well as to himself. There is a need for attention that is common in children this age.

There is a healthy balance between superego, ego, and id, with each being developed beyond what one would expect to find in the typical seven-year-old.

Jerry

There is a childlike quality in Jerry's handwriting that could be regarded as a becoming trait. Jerry is still in the process of *becoming* the total person he is capable of being. His strongest trait is his consistently optimistic attitude toward the future.

Emotional Structure. Perspectrograph # 2 shows Jerry to be much more emotionally responsive than Peter: 12% of Jerry's emotional structure is objective (AB), while 22% is moderately responsive (BC), 50% is very responsive (CD), and 16% is impulsive (DE). Jerry likes people and is responsive to people as well as to his environment.

Thinking Patterns. Jerry thinks in a plodding manner. He does not learn quickly nor easily but he learns thoroughly. He is somewhat creative in his thinking patterns and prefers logical concepts to abstract ones. He tends to be more analytical in his thinking than Peter: he wants to know the *why* as well as the *how*.

Personality Profile. Jerry exhibits the same ability to use his hands creatively as Peter. He shows fair ability to pay attention to detail as well as some organizational ability. He is quite generous to causes and people he believes are worthy. He tends to be practical in setting his goals but also shows some idealism. He has the necessary willpower to meet his goals, though occasionally he needs encouragement in this. He occasionally procrastinates. At times he becomes more determined to meet his goals when faced with adversity. He is an independent thinker at times.

Jerry is a very talkative person. He feels very protective about what he feels is his. He can be stubborn when pressed. He exhibits some self-control—possibly attempting to control his very optimistic attitude.

Jerry feels bad when criticized. There is a small indication of occasional temper.

Johnny

Johnny is a mercurial, restless, unpredictable person, quickly moving between being evasive, brutal, and at times conniving. He is a very "feeling" person.

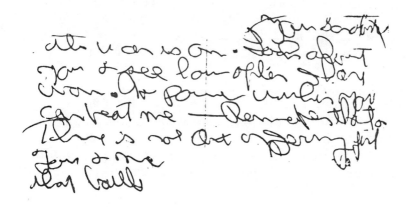

Emotional Structure. Perspectrograph #3 shows Johnny to be 4% withdrawn (FA), 24% objective (AB), 43% moderately responsive (BC), 17% very responsive (CD), 10% impulsive (DE), and 2% very impulsive (E+). Johnny moves quickly from one extreme to the other—from withdrawn to highly impulsive. He completely experiences the full range of emotions.

Thinking Patterns. Johnny thinks more quickly than Peter or Jerry and grasps concepts more rapidly. However, he does not pursue concepts to the depth that Peter and Jerry do. He prefers to skim the surface, grasping as much as he can as quickly as he can. He feels more comfortable with logical concepts and is adept at manipulating logic to his advantage.

Personality Profile. Johnny is a restless person who wants and needs to dominate situations and people. At times he is cruel to others. He likes responsibility and tends to guard it carefully. He is a talkative person and does not always use good judgment in his speech. However, a natural tendency to diplomacy often rescues him from difficult places his impulsiveness has taken him.

He likes to be involved in many activities and ideas and occasionally becomes confused in his thinking because of his many interests and needs.

Johnny is an independent thinker. There is very little of the generosity found in Peter and Jerry. Generosity is not a natural trait for Johnny but one he has acquired to use only when he feels it will gain something for him.

Johnny usually sets realistic goals but at times is idealistic in his goal-setting. When faced with adversity, he increases his willpower to help him attain his goals.

There is a considerable amount of stubbornness exhibited. He will not give in even when proved to be wrong.

Even though cruelty and evasiveness are exhibited, there is only one indication of temper shown in the available specimen of handwriting.

Johnny appears to recognize some of his weaknesses, as two indications of deliberate self-control are visible.

Most of Johnny's time and energy are directed toward trying to meet his many needs, by whatever means necessary.

Dana

Dana is objective, intuitive, and decisive. He is an ideal "problem solver."

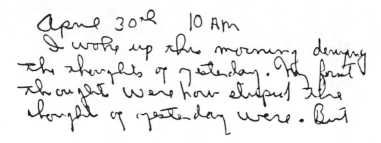

Emotional Structure. Perspectrograph #4 shows Dana to be 5% withdrawn (FA), 25% objective (AB), 49% moderately responsive (BC), 16% very responsive (CD), and 5% impulsive (DE). Dana is more objective than Johnny or Jerry. He is not especially withdrawn, nor is he overly impulsive. He is a cool, objective person who reacts to people with warmth and empathy but maintains his perspective at all times and makes decisions based on objective data.

Thinking Patterns. Dana exhibits a greater variety of thinking patterns than Peter, Jerry, or Johnny, indicating a higher intelligence. However, being able to think in a variety of ways often creates conflict for Dana. He has a greater ability to concentrate than the other three just described. He has creative as well as analytical thinking patterns present. Dana also has some intuition—a thinking pattern not found in the previous three. He is able to understand people and situations without always knowing how he knows. He has the ability to "sense" the feeling tone in a room occupied by people. Dana uses both his intuition and logic to obtain knowledge. Conflict appears when he must choose between logical solutions and intuitive knowledge.

Dana is highly analytical and questions a great deal. He is able to flow easily in his thinking, going comfortably from one train of thought to another.

Personality Profile. Once conflict is resolved by weighing available information, Dana is a very decisive person, able to make decisions quickly and with finality. He is the "problem solver" of the four.

Dana also exhibits the ability to work creatively with his hands. He is independent in his thinking and actions but can conform easily if it seems to the best advantage.

Dana finds that his ability to think in a variety of ways often causes him to procrastinate in taking action. However, once he starts on a course, he quickly assimilates information and makes decisions based on the information available.

Dana is a very good organizer and has the ability to take care of details.

He is very talkative but is always in control of what he is saying and is able to validate his statements. He likes to assume responsibility.

Dana is not as generous as Peter and Jerry. His actions of giving will be based on objective evaluations of the situation rather than on his own responsive feelings.

Dana is an idealist in setting his goals but has the necessary willpower to attain his goals. He has a very optimistic attitude.

He is direct in his approach to people and situations. When faced with adversity, he increases his effort to attain his goal. He can also be stubborn even when he knows that he may not be right. However, he is also sensitive to criticism from others.

Henry

Henry is more gentle in his nature than the previous four personalities described and has fewer defenses evident.

I am writing this as you requested. I
hope that all goes well in the sale of your
new book just on the shelves of the book
shelves. I haven't seen it yet. But I
will look in our local book stores in
the next couple of days

Emotional Structure. Perspectrograph #5 shows that 8% of Henry's emotional structure is objective (AB), 24% is moderately responsive (BC), 56% is very responsive (CD), and 12% is impulsive (DE). Henry's emotional structure is very similar to Jerry's. He is basically a warm, responsive person.

Thinking Patterns. Henry also thinks a great deal like Jerry. He uses the same thinking patterns, causing him to think in a creative manner and preferring not to be rushed.

Personality Profile. Henry tends to be idealistic in setting his goals and has a very optimistic attitude toward attaining them. He can be enthusiastic about things he enjoys. He shows organizational ability, some ability to notice and take care of details, and feels protective toward things and people belonging to him. Occasionally, he overlooks details he views as unimportant.

He is loyal to what he believes to be right. Henry welcomes responsibility and receives it with a conscientious attitude. He is also quite talkative.

Summary

There is sufficient evidence in graphological indicators for us to conclude that the five hands were written by one person—but that that one person contains different personalities.

There is a noticeable lack of rationalization exhibited in each of the five hands. In each case the ego faces situations in an honest, accepting way, rather than attempting to rationalize. The trait of rationalization is a common one found in many adult hands. It reveals one of the ego's methods of coping with uncomfortable life situations and relationships. It represents the ego's compromise between personal integrity and actual reality and results in a distorted view of reality. These five hands indicate personalities stubbornly refusing to compromise the self in uncomfortable life situations. Yet, the original basic personality felt a demanding need to split itself into several parts, or fragments, in order to pursue the growth of the whole until these conflicting emotional expressions could be unified into one growing, becoming-whole personality.

The stroke revealing talkativeness is found in many instances in each of the five hands but is not as prevalent in Henry's. The need for verbal expression appears to be somewhat reconciled through the four previous hands, so that the final handwriting of the patient does not show as much need for verbal expression of the personality. The fifth hand (Henry's) also exhibits considerably fewer defense mechanisms than the first four.

Dana's handwriting exhibits higher than normal intelligence, but the other four indicate personalities of average intelligence. However, there is a much greater amount of drive for achievement than is found in average handwriting. The fairly heavy pressure found in all five hands reveals personalities that absorb and retain experiences for long periods of time.

The final impression is one of a person of average intelligence (with the exception of Dana) and education but with superior drive, ambition, and optimism, combined with an honest outlook, who would not be denied in his search for wholeness nor be willing to compromise any of the self that is striving so hard to develop during all of this time.

Graphological Similarities

1. *Margins:* Margins in all five handwriting specimens

are similar. The same amount of space is left on the left margin in each sample of handwriting and the same amount of space is also left on the right margin. All five have wider left-hand margins than right-hand margins.

2. *Size:* All five specimens would be considered medium-sized handwriting, as measured on the Ana-Graph. The greatest variations are between Johnny's and Dana's, with Johnny's at times measuring somewhat larger than medium and Dana's occasionally measuring smaller than medium. A total stroke count reveals that all show a majority of medium-sized strokes.

3. *Pressure (depth):* The analyst worked with xerox copies of handwriting specimens from Peter, Jerry, Johnny, and Dana, and the original from Henry. Peter's handwriting sample had many of the characteristics of pencil writing. Jerry, Johnny, and Dana appear to have used a ballpoint pen for the handwriting or a very fine felt-tip pen. Henry's was written with a medium ball-point pen. All five specimens appear to be written with about the same degree of pressure. There is a greater degree of variance from light to dark shading in Peter's handwriting, possibly due to the pencil being used. Jerry's shows a consistent pressure. Dana's shows heavier pressure on downstrokes. Johnny's shows the greatest variance from light to dark shading in specimens where a ball-point pen was used. It is possible (but this is only speculation) that the samples from Jerry, Johnny, and Dana were all written with the same ball-point pen.

Henry's handwriting specimen is the only original and shows a heavy primary pressure applied with a medium ball-point pen. Xerox copies of Henry's handwriting reveal that it is consistent with the other copies, especially Jerry's.

4. *Zones:*

PETER—The *upper zones* contain some large upper loops in *h* letters. The other upper loops are average in size. The *middle zone* is distinct, well developed, and

rounded. The *lower zone* is well developed and propor-
tioned.

Total overview: The three zones are well balanced.

JERRY—The *upper zones* show some large *h* loops
with the rest being average in size. The *middle zone* is distinct, well developed, and rounded. The *lower zone* reveals
two with short endings, three with average-length endings.

Total overview: The three zones are well balanced.

JOHNNY—The *upper zones* contain some large *h* and
b and *k* loops. The *middle zone* is thready, receding, poorly
defined. There are two hooks shown in this zone. The *lower
zone* is not developed, is incomplete and distorted.

Total overview: There is unbalance. The development of
the id is incomplete. Emphasis is on the middle zone (daily
routine in living) while great imagination is shown in the
intellectual, or abstract, area.

DANA—In the *upper zone*, we find seven inflated
upper loops and fifteen average-sized upper loops. Several
of the *t*'s and *d*'s have short stems. The *middle zone* is not
as distinct as in Peter and Jerry but is well developed and
is average to small in size. In the *lower zone*, we find long
ending strokes in the *y*'s. These are incomplete, as the
stroke does not come back up to the baseline. There are
two "hooks" in the lower zone. The lower loops are narrow
in width. This, combined with the length, reveals a person
with a restless nature, who does not open himself to others
easily or quickly.

Total overview: The emphasis is on the upper and lower
zones. The middle zone is not as pronounced, indicating
that the superego and id are well developed while the ego
functions normally. Energy is directed to the subconscious
and the superego rather than to mundane, routine activities.

HENRY—The *upper zone* contains tall loops with
large inflated *h*'s and *k*'s. The upper zone is clear and well

defined. The *middle zone* is distinct, well developed, and rounded. The *lower zone* contains some incomplete lower stroke endings in the *y*'s. There are four quite long endings and ten average.

Total overview: The three zones are well balanced.

5. *Beginning Strokes:*

Short and curved: Peter 7, Johnny 3, Henry 10 (first 5 lines), Jerry 12, Dana 7.

Direct: Peter 3, Johnny 8, Henry 0, Jerry 5, Dana 6.

Hooks: Peter 0, Johnny 4, Henry 0, Jerry 0, Dana 2.

The following samples show beginning strokes that are consistent in all five hands:

Peter   Johnny   Henry

Jerry   Dana

Conclusions: The consistency of the beginning strokes in ratio to the number shown reveals that these were written by the same writer.

6. *Ending Strokes:*

Curved upward:
Peter—seven in first line. His ending strokes are consistently done in this manner.
Jerry—five in first line of writing.
Johnny—three in entire specimen (two are distorted).
Dana—none.
Blunt:
Peter—none.
Jerry—four in first three lines.

Johnny—eleven in first four lines.
Dana—ten in first four lines.
Henry—four in first two lines.

Conclusion: The consistency of the ending strokes in ratio to the number shown reveals that these were all made by the same writer.

7. *Connectedness:* Peter and Jerry have completely connected letters in words in the lower-case letters. Johnny has two breaks in words but the rest of the words have small letters connected. Dana has six breaks in words with the rest connected. Henry has one break in the first five lines.

Conclusion: The consistency of breaks within words in ratio to the number of words written reveals that these were all made by the same writer.

8. *Spacing between letters:* The letters *th* were used for measurement. The space measured was at the middle of the bottom of the letter *t* to the upstroke on *h*.

Peter	Three had a space of two millimeters
	Two had a space of two and one half millimeters
	Five had a space of three millimeters
Jerry	Three had a space of three millimeters
Johnny	One had a space of two millimeters
	One had a space of three millimeters
	One had a space of five millimeters
Dana	One had a space of two millimeters
	One had a space of five millimeters
	Three had a space of three mi¹limeters
	Two had a space of four millimeters
Henry	Three had a space of three millimeters
	One had a space of two millimeters
	Three had a space of four millimeters

Conclusions: The consistency of the size of the space between letters measured in ratio to the number available reveals that three millimeters was the average and that all five hands were done by the same writer.

9. *Spacing between words:* There was a variance from two to seven millimeters found in all five hands.

Conclusion: The consistency of the variance in spacing indicates that all five hands were made by the same writer.

10. *Flat-topped r:* This graphological indicator reveals the ability to work well with the hands. This is not a common trait frequently found in handwriting. It would be an impossible coincidence for this to appear in five separate hands. It appears consistently enough in these five to be considered evidence that the five samples were written by the same writer.

Samples: Peter - 18   Johnny - 1

Jerry - 4   Dana - 4   Henry - 10

11. *Beginning circle loops:* These were found in all five hands.

Samples: Peter   Johnny   Henry

Jerry   Dana

12. *Open-circle letters:*   This includes *o*'s and *a*'s, with a
flat horizontal stroke extending to the right.

Samples: Peter - 4   Johnny - 3   Henry - 8 (first 8 lin

Jerry - 6   Dana - 6

13. *T's and d's with "tend"-type base:*

Samples: Peter - 7   Johnny - 5   Henry - 3

Jerry - 5   Dana - 7

14. *Downward-curved t bars:*

Samples: Peter - 4   Johnny - 2   Henry - 2

Jerry - 1   Dana - 1

15. *Short t and d stems:*

Samples: Peter - 7   Johnny - 4   Henry - 5

16. *Balanced f:*

Samples: Peter - 4   Johnny - none   Henry - 4

Jerry - 1   Dana - 2

17. *Beginning stroke absent on w:*

Samples: Peter - 1   Johnny - 4   Henry - none

Jerry - 2   Dana - 5

18. *Similar capital R and B:*

Samples: Peter - 4   Johnny - 1   Henry

Jerry - none   Dana - 1

19. *Capital I with base missing:*

Samples: Peter - none   Johnny - 3   Henry - 1

Jerry - none   Dana - 4

20. *Small b with no beginning stroke:*

Samples: Peter - 2   Johnny - 3   Henry - none

Jerry - 3   Dana - 2

21. *Large, inflated h loops:*

Samples: Peter - 9   Johnny - 6   Henry - 7 (first 4

Jerry - 5   Dana - 5

Other: Capital *A* in Peter's and Dana's hands has same broad base with narrow top.

Samples: Peter   Dana

Personality Similarities

1. *Temper:*   Peter - 7   Johnny - 1   Henry - 2
(slight)   Jerry - 1   Dana - 3

2. *Procrastination:*   Peter - none   Johnny - 1
    Henry - 1   Jerry - 2   Dana - 4

3. *Stubbornness:*   Peter - 3   Johnny - 7   Henry - 5
Jerry - 3   Dana - 6

4. *Self-control:*   Peter - 1   Johnny - 2   Henry - 1
(very slight)   Jerry - 1   Dana - 1

5. *Sensitive to criticism:*   Peter - 4 (slight)   Johnny - 4
(moderate)   Jerry - 3 (slight)   Dana - 7
(slight)   Henry - 7 (slight)
                    25 (not sensitive)

6. *Idealistic goals:*   Peter - 13   Johnny - 3
Henry - 3   Jerry - 6   Dana - 9

7. *Generosity:*   Peter - 7   Johnny - 3   Henry - 4
(first 4 lines)   Jerry - 5   Dana - 1

8. *Logical thinking:*   Peter - completely logical
                    Johnny - predominantly logical
                    Jerry - completely logical
                    Dana - predominantly logical with
                    intuition present
                    Henry - predominantly logical

9. *Ability to use hands well:*   Peter - 18   Johnny - 1
Henry - 10   Jerry - 4   Dana - 4

10. *Welcomes responsibility:*   Peter - 1   Johnny - 1
Henry - 2   Jerry - 1   Dana - 1

11. *Jealousy:*   Peter - 3   Johnny - 3   Henry - 1
Jerry - 1   Dana - 0

12. *Talkative:*   Peter - 4   Johnny - 3   Henry - 8
Jerry - 6   Dana - 6

13. *Independent:*   Peter - 7   Johnny - 4   Henry - 5
Jerry - 3   Dana - 4

14. *Organizational ability:*   Peter - 4   Johnny -
none   Henry - 4   Jerry - 1   Dana - 2

15. *Direct:*   Peter - 3   Johnny - 7   Henry -
none   Jerry - 5   Dana - 7

16. *Good imagination:*   Peter - 9   Johnny - 6
Henry - 7   Jerry - 5   Dana - 5

NOTE: The number beside the name indicates the number of times this particular indicator is found in the sample. The numbers do not provide a valid comparison basis because the content of the writings is not the same. Some of the specimens are longer than others and some contain more of one particular letter than the others. The value of recording them is to show that the indicator is present in each of the writings rather than to give a comparison. This applies to both Personality Similarities and Graphological Similarities.

Graphological Differences

The greatest difference is in the slant of each hand, which indicates the emotional responsiveness of each writer. The Perspectrographs provide visual illustrations of this. Jerry and Henry are very similar in emotional structure. Johnny, Peter, and Dana have similar emotional structures. The greatest difference is between Henry and Peter.

Peter is the only writer who uses the circle i dot in his writing and it is found only once. The circle i dot is quite common in the handwriting of children.

Each of the five samples would be considered medium in size but the greatest variance is between Johnny and Dana. Some of Johnny's strokes would be considered large while a portion of Dana's would be considered small. However, the average of the total is still medium.

Personality Differences

The traits of temper, stubbornness, and undeveloped self-concept are consistently found in the writing of Peter, Jerry, Johnny, and Dana, but are seen much less in the writing of Henry. While these traits are present in Henry's writing, they are not found to the degree that they are found in the others.

The capital I is one indicator of ego development. There is no capital I in Peter's handwriting so his ego development cannot be evaluated on that basis.

The missing base on the capital I with a rounded top indicates incomplete ego development. More of these were found in the writing of Johnny and Dana. The capital I's found in the writing of Peter, Jerry, and Henry show more complete I's. In Henry's writing, one is found without a base while six are completed. This indicates an ego growth and development present in Henry's writing that is lacking (in various degrees) in the other four.

Personality Emphasis

Peter personality—creativity, balance, objectivity
Jerry personality—prevailing hopeful attitude, helpful
Johnny personality—avenue for feelings (predominantly negative)
Dana personality—problem solver, unifier, objective, ability to understand other personalities and work with them.